GOOD DOCTORS, GOOD PATIENTS: PARTNERS IN HIV TREATMENT

JUDITH G. RABKIN, PhD, MPH
ROBERT H. REMIEN, PhD
CHRISTOPHER R. WILSON, RN, MPH

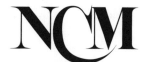

NCM

PUBLISHERS, INC.

New York, New York
1994

*To Lewis Katoff, Ph.D., our friend, our colleague,
and our partner in research, who was there from the beginning
and whose example continues to inspire us.*

The drugs, medical approaches, recommendations, procedures, and anecdotes included in this book are intended to educate, inspire, and supplement—not replace—the medical advice of a trained healthcare professional. All health matters should be discussed with an appropriate practitioner. A physician should be consulted before any medicinal agent or procedure is adopted. This book represents the opinions of the authors and does not necessarily reflect the opinions of the publishers or the institutions with which the authors are affiliated.

© 1994 by NCM Publishers, Inc.
All rights reserved. Printed in the United States of America. No part of this book may be reproduced in any manner without written permission. Address inquiries to NCM Publishers, Inc., 200 Varick Street, New York, NY 10014.

Library of Congress Catalog Card Number 94-74840
ISBN: 0-9643884-0-5

This book is printed on recycled paper.

CONTENTS

ACKNOWLEDGEMENTS

Partial support was provided by:

American Suicide Foundation

Roerig, a Division of Pfizer Pharmaceuticals, Inc.
(educational grant)

HIV Center for Clinical and Behavioral Studies,
N.Y. State Psychiatric Institute

Burroughs Wellcome Co. (educational grant)

We wish to thank the doctors and patients who participated in the study interviews and shared their experience and knowledge with us, as well as our editor, Margie Miller, and the staff at NCM Publishers, Inc. who helped us translate our thoughts into print.

The following people reviewed part or all of the manuscript and provided valuable feedback and suggestions:

Marina Alvarez
Lisa Capaldini, M.D.
David Gold
Damien Kimpton, M.S.T.
Laura Pinsky, M.S.W.
Michael Shernoff, M.S.W.
Peter Ungvarski, M.S., R.N.
Dan William, M.D.

WE REMEMBER THE LIVES OF

Charles Barber
Michael Callen
Tom Cunningham
Eric Kendrick
James Lamphear
Aldyn McKean
Robert McMenemy
Leon McKusick, Ph.D.
Michael Marshall
Dann O'Connor
Robert Perantoni
Jim Serafini, Ph.D.

PREFACE

"I'm completely different than I was prior to getting sick.
I'm much more who I always wanted to be,
who I always imagined I'd be.
I just didn't know when to begin getting serious about my life.
AIDS has made that very clear."

These are the words of a long-term AIDS survivor, reflecting on his life before and after diagnosis. Our lives, too, have been changed by AIDS. This book represents much of what we have learned through our collective experiences—about life in general and about life with HIV. More specifically, we have come to realize that a fierce and independent will to live, combined with health-enhancing behaviors and talented, compassionate physicians, can contribute to prolonged survival. Even when cure is not possible, a life of quality and value can be sustained until the end. And when the struggle is almost over, even death can be handled well.

We can't see life the way we used to see it, nor are we sure we would want to, despite the tragedy and losses that have been part of the process. It has altered the way we think about living and dying, health and sickness, curing and healing, and what each of those concepts really means. We have been reminded that healing is not always the same as curing. We've had to learn how to incorporate the sorrow and anger, and sometimes despair, that are inevitable components of being close to people with and living with HIV. At the same time, our lives have been immeasurably enriched.

Under normal circumstances, it is usually the elderly who have a true sense of death as an integral part of life. Now, thanks to our intense—and often agonizing—experiences with continued loss, we, too, have achieved a kind of accelerated wisdom and recognition of the fragility and value of life. It is perhaps the ultimate irony that a renewed passion for living has been born from the devastation of AIDS.

Sitting by the bedsides of sick friends, we have seen how they've worked with their doctors in both positive and negative ways. We have learned firsthand how the quality and even length of life can be influenced by the doctor-patient relationship. We've also seen how caring friends and family can infuse life with meaning, despite illness.

We have experienced the helplessness of waiting for answers that are too slow in coming, waiting for medical cures for diseases whose names were, until recently, unknown. We've waited for hours with a frightened and worried patient for the physician to return a telephone call. We've held the hand of a friend who was dying, reassured by the competence of a coordinated home care team and the comfort of a compassionate physician.

Although there is yet no cure for AIDS, our experiences have shown us what can be done, and done well, by those caught up in the struggle. Moreover, while we recognize that relationships between patients and their physicians can be as variable and complex as any, a good match can result in prolonged and healthier survival.

We've also been inspired by patients, their families, and their physicians, just as patients, families, and physicians are often inspired by each other. Their loyalty, affection, and attachments have been a testimony to the resilience and strength of ordinary people facing difficult times.

What we've tried to capture in this book are some of the lessons we have learned from patients and doctors, about patients and doctors, in both research and clinical settings. We draw on our collective professional and personal experiences in formal research, clinical service, volunteer work, and supervision and training since 1984. Between 1990 and 1994, we conducted a study of nearly 100 men and women long-term AIDS survivors—the AIDS Long-Term Survivor Study. As part of that study, we interviewed 25 physicians in New York City and San Francisco who were identified as outstanding AIDS specialists by other physicians, AIDS community organizations, and patients. We sought to determine what maintains hope, what diminishes hope, and what leads to a loss of hope among people with AIDS. We also wanted to learn whether certain personal qualities, attitudes, and medical strategies are associated with longer survival. What we discovered from this illuminating process has been incorporated throughout this book, often in the words of "survivors" and physicians themselves.

Cumulatively, we have published over 150 papers in professional journals and books, as well as community publications. We have lectured at national and international professional conferences and federal hearings and have given informal talks at workshops and community meetings. We have visited our patients and our friends at home and in the hospital; we have seen illness and recovery from illness; we have attended memorial services; and we have participated in the process of "healing." Our intention here is to lead others involved in this plague to a sense of healing.

New York City   —*Judith G. Rabkin*
December 1994   —*Robert H. Remien*
                                                            —*Christopher R. Wilson*

INTRODUCTION

A IDS is a unique disease with specific as well as universal challenges for physicians and patients. As with other chronic illnesses, over the years, the primary doctor-patient relationship can take on singular significance, providing constancy and comfort in a life too often filled with uncertainty and crisis. For people with AIDS (PWAs), the association with a caring physician may constitute one of the patient's most enduring and emotionally intimate connections. Success can mean a fruitful interaction, in which patient and physician share expectations, communicate well, and feel satisfied about their collaboration at all stages of illness up to and including the patient's death, should that occur. A failed relationship, on the other hand, can lead to hostility, frustration, and demoralization; it can also result in inadequate or inappropriate medical care.

In the course of our work as clinicians and researchers, we have been impressed with the apparently crucial role of the doctor-patient relationship in maintaining the well-being and health of people with HIV. Medical management of this difficult and complicated illness requires extraordinary dedication and effort on the part of both physician and patient, as well as skills not often found in the repertoire of most people.

AIDS specialists are constantly confronted with crises. They face demands that require immense flexibility, tolerance, and an ability to suspend their primary identity as "one who cures." One physician explained that he conceives of AIDS as a long and difficult war, in which he won many battles except the last. Even then, he noted, when death is handled compassionately, according to the patient's wishes, that, too, can be a sort of victory.

PWAs also are confronted with recurrent crises and decisions, and they, too, face demands that require flexibility, initiative, and the courage not to "follow the rules." Hallmarks of the "good" HIV patient include realism and pragmatism, as well as both the willingness and the capacity to take charge of his or her own health by being a good medical consumer. The patient and the physician must make difficult treatment decisions that make sense to both. Since such decisions are usually carried out without the reassurance of scientific data, psychologically, this is no small challenge. Paradoxically, the patient must allow him- or herself to experience a full range of emotions, including depression and fear, while not giving in to despair. It is this balancing of hope and realism that presents a unique challenge to the patient living with HIV infection.

THE LONG HAUL

In a curious way, effective HIV physicians and patients often resemble each other, sharing crucial qualities that include not only the ability to act in a crisis but also persistence, tolerance for ambiguity, and endurance. In the heat of "battle," it is easy to mobilize energy, effort, and courage. It is the long haul that is truly difficult.

On the 50th anniversary of D-day, an old soldier wrote an essay about the war and his subsequent life:

> "Wear the silver badge of courage, drop like an eagle on your prey," the airborne recruiting posters had said. I jumped into Normandy a few hours before dawn on D-day. I was there in Holland and the Battle of the Bulge. [For many years I believed] that taking part in those campaigns with the 82nd Airborne Division overshadowed all that followed, including love, marriage, career, and children. That is no longer true. I have belatedly come to understand that slogging across the plain of everyday life with dignity and as much honesty as one can muster calls for as much heroism, if only because the struggle never ends, as does assaulting a flaming hill. (Bryant N. When the old wound aches. *The New York Times*. 1994, June 5, Section 4, p 1).

As this soldier has realized, valor is demonstrated not only on the battlefield but on the "plain of everyday life." The true challenge of HIV illness lies not only in medical crises but also in the days and months of uncertainty, of low-grade symptoms, discomfort, slow losses, deaths of friends, the exigencies of living daily with ambiguous but probably progressive decline. The definition of "grace under pressure" has to be extended beyond the sudden crisis to include the pressures of facing an illness of unknown nature and uncertain course. The effect of AIDS on the human body is ultimately devastating. The effect of AIDS on the human spirit can be transforming and inspirational.

THE CHANGING CLIMATE OF HOPE

News Conference, 1984

Health and Human Services Secretary Margaret Heckler confidently predicted at a Washington news conference: "There will be a vaccine in a very few years, and a cure for AIDS before 1990."

Time Magazine, December, 1986

The first effective anti-AIDS vaccines could come into use by 1990 at the earliest, WHO officials believe. (*Time*. 1986, December 1, p 45)

Cover Line, *Body Positive*, 1988

My guess is that within 12 to 18 months, we will be able to arrest the disease at whatever stage it's at, except for people who are extremely sick. Also by that time we will be able to begin to restore immune function back toward normal (Bernard Bihari, MD. *Body Positive*. 1988, February, Cover).

Advertisement for *Time Magazine*, 1992

In the mid-1980's, scientists believed a vaccine for AIDS would be ready in two years. Seven years later: no vaccine, no cure, no reliable treatment. With over 250,000 dead and another 272,000 living with AIDS, no American will escape the effects of this century's most deadly disease. Which is why this wasn't the first time, nor the last, you'll find AIDS on the cover of *Time*.

Op-ed Column, *The New York Times*, 1992

Title: "Don't Bet on a Miracle." Text: Why...does the future look so bleak? The answer is that given what we know today, it cannot be predicted when, or even if, an effective treatment will be developed and when, or if, a vaccine will be developed (William Haseltine, MD, Chief of Human Retrovirology, Harvard University. *The New York Times*. 1992, November 15, p A55).

Cover, *The New York Times Magazine*, 1993

I am getting sicker. Time is running out. Once AIDS was a hot topic. But now the world is moving on, uncaring, frustrated and bored, leaving by the roadside those of us who are infected and who can't help but wonder, "Whatever happened to AIDS?" (Jeffrey Schmalz, *New York Times* reporter and PWA, *The New York Times Magazine*. 1993, November 28). [Since Schmalz was still working on this article when he died, it turned out to be his obituary as well as yet another "call to arms."]

The Nation, July 4, 1994

The AIDS problem of these times has very little to do with an uncaring world or a conspiracy of silence. Hardest is acknowledging that AIDS is not a transitory phenomenon—a momentary disaster that will be stopped by scientists who, in their quest for the Nobel Prize, will come up with the magic bullet. The hope early on was that HIV would, like polio, be tamed by knowledge, but the fact is that HIV is much more like cancer, stubbornly resistant to the ingenuity of scientists. (Kirp D. After the band stopped playing. *The Nation*. 1994, July 4, pp 14-17).

There is a paradox among physicians, researchers, patients, and the general public in their collective perceptions about the management of AIDS. Major strides have been made in the basic sciences. We understand more about HIV and about how to treat specific opportunistic infections. An array of at least partly effective antiretroviral agents has been marketed since 1987. Nevertheless, expectations regarding cure and survival, at least for the near future, are more modest now than they were 5 years ago. Perhaps as a consequence, AIDS has received less attention in the media (major newspapers and newsweeklies) in 1994 than in any year since 1986 (*Time*, August 22, 1994, p15).

AN HISTORICAL PERSPECTIVE

During the first years of the epidemic, arbitrarily defined as between 1981 and 1984, there was usually no warning of impending illness. People often discovered their illness for the first time in the emergency room when an AIDS-defining condition was diagnosed. Before 1986, HIV testing was not generally available, except to a handful of people enrolled in studies in which blood samples were sent to Europe for testing. Until mid-1987, when AZT was first marketed, many gay advocacy organizations opposed HIV testing because the risks of confirming HIV seropositivity (in terms of distress and possible discrimination) were considered to outweigh any benefits. In essence, without an early warning system, there was no practical way to "prepare" for illness.

There were no established treatments for AIDS-defining conditions, and no physicians who were "AIDS specialists." In those early days, it was difficult to admit sick HIV patients into hospitals; hospital staffs were often hostile, and there was very little formal or informal professional support for physicians who treated HIV patients.

As one physician recalled, "In the early days of the epidemic, I felt much more estranged and isolated. In those days you were sort of winging it, with very little information or support. We had very few interventions, and we didn't know what the hell was going on. My first case of AIDS in 1980 kept me up at night, gave me cramps and insomnia, and made me feel inept, impotent, and worthless."

By the mid-1980s, the epidemic, together with supportive services, had grown to the extent that there were sufficient numbers of affected people (patients and helpers) to begin to speak of an AIDS community. At the end of 1985, the HIV-antibody test became commercially available, and gradually, increasing numbers of middle-class people in high-risk groups learned of their HIV status long before they actually became ill. [It is unfortunately still true that too many men and women in poor urban communities continue to be unaware of their HIV-positive status until an emergency hospital admission, when an AIDS-defining condition is diagnosed.] Effective treatments were being developed for specific opportunistic infections. The prevailing belief during the mid-1980s was that while this was a crisis and people were dying, a cure would soon be discovered.

The availability of AZT in 1987 marked the beginning of a new era. Prophylaxis for *Pneumocystis carinii* pneumonia (PCP) became widespread and effective. A number of new and powerful treatments for other opportunistic infections were subsequently approved, including ganciclovir (Cytovene) for cytomegalovirus (CMV) retinitis, fluconazole (Diflucan) for other fungal infections, clarithromycin (Biaxin) and azithromycin (Zithromax) for *Mycobacterium avium intracellulare* complex (MAI), and recombinant colony–stimulating factors (erythropoietin [Procrit, Epogen] and filgrastrim [Neupogen]) for anemia and neutropenia, respectively. Additional antiretrovirals (ddI [didanosine, Videx], ddC [zalcitabine, Hivid], d4T [stavudine, Zerit]) have been recently approved, although their comparative efficacy remains unclear. Thus, treatment of infections and cancers has become more sophisticated and far more effective in the last 15 years, contributing significantly to an overall improvement in prognosis for PWAs.

There is little question that both physicians and patients have considerably different attitudes in the 1990s than in earlier years about prospects for health and survival after diagnosis of an AIDS-defining condition. Before 1987, for example, many patients were told that they had only 6 months to a year to live. This has changed. An AIDS diagnosis no longer means imminent demise to informed patients and health providers, although some members of the general public, and even some members of the gay community, continue to equate HIV with death. Declining suicide rates (1987-1989) among people with AIDS may also reflect greater optimism among PWAs about both quality of life and survival.

A new and vastly encouraging concept introduced at the 1994 International AIDS Conference is that of the "long-term non-progressor." This rather cumbersome phrase refers to people whose HIV seropositive status has been established unequivocably yet who remain immunologically healthy (CD4 cells >600 cells/cu.mm) and physically asymptomatic for 12 years or longer (definition according to David Ho, MD, 1994). Intensive study of such individuals may yield valuable information about protective factors of the host, or characteristics of certain viral strains, that may some day be used to develop prophylactic and/or therapeutic strategies for "progressors." The phenomenon of long-term non-progressors provides a tantalizing clue about the possibility of co-existence with HIV.

Nevertheless, most knowledgeable people, including physicians and patients, are not optimistic about the likelihood of a cure in time to save those already ill, nor is an effective vaccine yet on the horizon (as of late 1994). The hopelessness of the early years was first replaced by optimism about cure, which has now shifted to a more cautious expectation of incremental progress that will take many years to achieve.

AIDS MEDICINE AS A MODEL

The gravity of HIV illness, rapidly evolving treatment strategies, the changing conditions of the illness itself, and the politicized climate in which research, treatment, and funding issues are considered are some of the factors that color the task of AIDS specialists and AIDS patients and the way they work together. The study of the medical management of AIDS has unique elements in that it is a "new" disease with a definable chronological onset. Moreover, the first community afflicted in this country included a particularly educated and articulate group whose refusal to accept the traditional patient role constituted a departure from the conventional doctor-patient relationship. Finally, AIDS is one of the most complicated and difficult diseases ever identified, and its study at both the basic and clinical levels draws on biomedical techniques that did not even exist a decade ago. The relationships between PWAs and their physicians can be uniquely intense, given the chronicity and fatality of the disease, and the uncertainties of its manifestation and course.

But the medical management of AIDS and the evolving roles of AIDS doctors and AIDS patients also have implications for other areas of medicine and research. Women concerned about breast cancer have become interested in the consumer strategies of AIDS organizations, not only in terms of efforts to influence allocation of federal research and treatment funds but also in terms of educating patients about mastery skills associated with their medical care. A small but meaningful example concerns the wearing of a loop of red ribbon to signify "AIDS awareness" throughout 1992. Since then, the concept has caught on, with pink loops of ribbon signifying "breast cancer awareness."

What has been learned about doctor-patient relationships; about communication; about progressive illness; about how to manage living and dying with AIDS; and about preserving a sense of control, dignity, and privacy has general implications for a broad spectrum of physicians and patients. The strategies and approaches developed by experts in the context of AIDS medicine are particularly interesting for anyone who has or treats a chronic, life-threatening illness.

PURPOSE
The purpose of this book is to provide for patients, their loved ones, and the professionals and volunteers who work with people with HIV illness some understanding of the characteristics of effective physicians and effective patients. Moreover, we explore the mysteries of the doctor-patient relationship and how it may contribute to longevity. We examine what experienced physicians and experienced patients expect of themselves and each other, how they conceptualize their individual and joint responsibilities, how they communicate with each other, how they negotiate treatment plans and goals for living and sometimes for dying.

SOURCES
The material in this book is based on our cumulative clinical and research experience with several hundred patients. In addition, we conducted formal interviews with "AIDS experts" as part of a long-term survivor study over the past several years. By AIDS experts, we mean patients who are AIDS "long-term survivors," physicians who have large HIV/AIDS practices and have been involved since early in the epidemic, and other professionals with a wide range of experience in AIDS care, including nurses, clergy, counselors, patient educators, and advocates.

DEFINITIONS
An AIDS long-term survivor, as defined by the Centers for Disease Control and Prevention (CDC), is anyone living more than 3 years following diagnosis of an AIDS-defining opportunistic infection (not including Kaposi's sar-

coma)(1987 criteria). As of 1990, this was twice the median survival period (18 months) for gay men. Data indicate that 3-year survival rates for those diagnosed in the late 1980s fall into the 15% to 20% range. Most of those we interviewed were gay men since they were the first group diagnosed with AIDS and were the most identifiable "long-term survivors" when we began our research. Others include men and women living with HIV infection for many years, with or without symptoms. People who are HIV-positive but asymptomatic are referred to as "long-term non-progressors."

WHAT DOES THIS BOOK COVER?

This book presents the opinions of HIV-positive patients and their physicians, often in their own words, about what they believe to be the important characteristics of the "good" or successful patient and physician, the nature of the doctor-patient relationship, and the expectations each has of the other. These are lessons from "the frontline," gleaned from life, the hard way.

We recognize that other health providers actively contribute to the management of HIV illness: nurses, social workers, counselors, home care attendants, case managers, clergy, and hospice staff. Especially with progressive illness when patients require extended care, they may play important if not central roles. We focus here on the doctor-patient dyad not because it exists in a vacuum but because if it isn't a functioning relationship, nothing else can really take its place. We see it as the linchpin in the process of living and dying with AIDS.

While aware of cultural differences, we do not systematically address the impact of specific cultures or ethnicities in the pursuit of medical care. Similarly, we recognize that poverty, limited personal and social resources, and health care discrimination exist and influence HIV management. However, in this book we focus on issues of general relevance for anyone involved in AIDS care. Moreover, the perspectives offered in this book are those of "Western" medicine. All of the interviews conducted were with people, of diverse ethnic backgrounds, who receive or provide "western medical care." Other approaches to treatment are discussed within this context.

We discuss the medical and psychological challenges faced throughout the spectrum of HIV disease, from initial diagnosis up to and including end-stage disease and the dying process, if that is the outcome. This book describes specific skills and strategies to meet these challenges. We also discuss the "ups and downs," the rewards, and positive aspects of living with HIV and working with this population, as well as the negative consequences. Our focus is on the adult patient and his or her medical and social world. In addition, we briefly discuss the role of friends, family, and professional counselors in the ongoing challenge of living with HIV and AIDS.

WHO SHOULD READ THIS BOOK?

We hope that anyone who is living with HIV, or who cares about someone living with HIV, as well as health care providers and counselors who are working or thinking about working with people living with HIV and their care-partners, friends or family, will find this book helpful.

REFERENCE

Long-term non-progressors. Tenth International Conference on AIDS; Yokohama, Japan; August 7-12, 1994. Plenary Session 10.

1

"BILL"—GOOD PATIENT OR BAD PATIENT?

COMMENT

The following is an abbreviated transcript of an interview conducted in April 1990 as part of our Long-Term Survivor Study. A standardized semi-structured interview was intended, but it soon became apparent that Bill wanted to tell his story his way. Bill's thoughts about his life, his illness, and its medical management are, in a way, representative of the typical fears and frustrations experienced by people with AIDS. We hope that by presenting his story, in his own words, we can come closer to understanding the effects of this disease.

Bill was a 38-year-old writer, literary translator, and teacher with a graduate degree. He came from a Roman Catholic family and was raised in the western United States. He had lived alone for 8 years and was supported by the mother of a former student. He had no government benefits. It should be noted that this story spans the early years of the epidemic.

MEDICAL HISTORY

Q. Tell me about your AIDS diagnosis.

A. I knew in 1981 that I was diagnosed with leukopenia and swollen lymph glands. So my first awareness that something was wrong was in 1981. In 1982, I joined one of the earliest monitoring studies of gay men in New York, which was run at Mt. Sinai Hospital. I did it for two reasons. One was that I was in no frame of mind and never have been in the frame of mind to lie to myself about the possibility of something being wrong in my life. I wasn't afraid of it really. I would rather know than not know about everything. So, for selfish reasons, I could have my blood drawn and monitored and analyzed and pored over and graphed for free. Second, I just thought that it was incumbent on me if I could help in terms of research and learning that I should do it. I had been in the hepatitis study as well. I just believed at the time that it was my duty as a citizen to participate in those types of scientific studies. I feel very differently now. And I would never participate in any official scientific research ever again because my experience over the last 8 years has left such a terrible taste in my mouth.

Q. *So you're not involved in any of those studies anymore?*

A. No. I have almost nothing to do with official science any more. Almost all of my current medical regimen and strategies are derived from underground or community or alternative-based sources. But getting back to the medical history, I was fine except for severe lymphadenopathy and leukopenia through 1984. It wasn't until May of 1985 that I really started having problems. I was having problems with an incessant vertigo, inability to focus, and an uncontrollable left side. I was actually tripping in the street. And it took my doctor the better part of 1985 to do something about it. And, of course, it was toxoplasmosis, but it didn't get bad enough because you almost have to die before official science will intervene. It wasn't until I had a brain abscess in the upper right lobe in early 1986 that I was hospitalized. And after all those years of monitoring and going to doctors and knowing that I had this virus—which of course they only found out about in 1983—I was in the hospital and I got the CDC seal of approval on my version of what they call AIDS.

Q. *When did that occur?*

A. Early 1986. And then things started happening fast and furious. By 1987, I had KS [Kaposi's sarcoma]. I had these spots on my legs in very early 1987. They biopsied them three times. The first two times, they came back negative. And it took them 6 months. So, if you asked a doctor when I became sick with KS, they would tell you it was at the end of 1987. That's a lie. I had KS early in 1987. I held my own fairly well until the end of 1988 when I started having serious gastrointestinal problems, which worsened throughout 1989. Finally, I had an endoscopy done, and in 1989, I had piled on me a diagnosis of KS of the intestines, CMV [cytomegalovirus] of the ileum, MAI [*Mycobacterium avium intracellulare* complex] of the ileum, and general AIDS wasting syndrome. At the end of 1989, they hooked me up to DHPG [ganciclovir] for quite a while to treat the CMV. All of this, of course, made me worse than I'd been before, and by November of 1989, I was dying. I was lying on my couch wasting, completely dehydrated and unable to eat anything at all. On an absorption study scale of 1 to 20, I was absorbing food only at about 7, which is technical starvation. But I'm doing better now because I've been taking compound Q on my own. Well, not on my own. I had assistance from a medical professional, but she only monitors me after I've already had the infusion.

TAKING CHARGE CREATIVELY: LYING, CHEATING, STEALING

Q. *How often have you done compound Q?*

A. I've been doing it according to the protocol they used in California. I mean I haven't run out and found vials and shot them into my veins. The saga of how I even came to be able to have the infusions of compound Q is just another one of these typical struggles of people trying to get the medical establishment to help them live and running into every conceivable road-block. But I had obtained a copy of the Project Inform protocol, as early as August of 1989, so that I knew what I needed in terms of equipment and that sort of thing. Getting a medical professional to help me out with it, however, was another story. So, I simply had it administered beginning in December, several weeks before Christmas. The first two infusions were 1 week apart at escalating dosages, starting out quite low. Based on the information that Project Inform had submitted to the FDA, I knew that I was at a high risk for central nervous system reaction. And so, rather than just pump the whole vial of this stuff into me, I spoke with doctors, I spoke with people in San Francisco who had helped administer compound Q. I read Asian medical journals about compound Q and decided on a very low dose the first time and increased it the second time a week later. There was a month between the third and fourth infusions, which I just had a week ago last Saturday. Last week was extremely brutal and culminated in my first real full-blown central nervous system reaction. I'm going to have a CAT scan and whatnot this week to be able to proceed with the next infusion with the maximum amount of information and as much certainty as possible that it's reasonably safe to go on.

But back to the compound Q episode and what it took. Let's see, I started in May of 1989. By September, my doctor had agreed in principle to do it. But Gina Kolata's [science writer] hatchet job [Sept 19, section C, p 1] on compound Q came out in *The New York Times* at that very time. I think it was September 17th and my doctor, although I had been feeding him all the information from the Miami study of course, hadn't read any of it, hadn't even looked at it. In fact, he gets all of his information about AIDS from *The New York Times*. Anyway, I had the first copy of the Miami study in New York, all of the Asian medical journal articles, all the Project Inform protocols and everything else. And the doctor called me and crapped out on me. When I asked him, "You mean you would rather that I did this alone here at home?" he said, "Yes." And I said to myself, this man is not the person that I should be seeing. And I was left high and dry with the compound Q and had to start looking again. Then the one doctor in New York who I knew could help me, stonewalled me, even though I had patients of hers talk to her privately on my behalf. Finally, I found someone in November and we started in December. Of course, that was all predicated on me having all of the filter needles; all of the tubing; all of the I.V. bags; all of the epinephrine and the antihistamine in case of an anaphylactic reaction, an allergic reaction; having all of the dexamethasone on hand, and of course, the syringes. That was all entirely up to me. Every piece of apparatus, everything was up to me. To protect the medical professional, who finally was brave enough to say that I would be monitored, we've been extremely careful about the fact that I open the vial, I provide the Q. I open the bottle of Q with a stone glass cutter from the doctor's office. I measure it out, I insert it into that bag, and I hook up the I.V. tubing to the bag and to a heplock, which is put in my arm by a nurse who sneaks away from her daily rounds and comes whenever I need her to do this simply as a favor, again risking her position and her job to do it. She was risking her position and, yet, it's the only thing that has ever been done for me of real worth, of real human seriousness throughout this whole thing.

So, that's a sort of thumbnail sketch of the latest Q thing, but I was already smuggling ribavirin from Mexico in 1985 and making AL-721. I forged a pathology report from Cabrini [hospital] in 1986. Of course, it was one of their botched KS pathology reports, and I doctored it, so to speak, until I had what basically amounted to a blank form with all of the characteristic numbers and the signature of the pathologist and whatnot. Although I had now been given the CDC seal of approval for my version of the disease, at the end of 1986, they were going to start providing AZT in the first generalized study but only to those people who had PCP [*Pneumocystis carinii* pneumonia]. Now, any moron knows that AZT was not treating PCP, that AZT actually deals with the underlying problem which all AIDS patients share: reverse transcriptase in the virus once it enters the cell. Of course, only those who had the same version of the disease, the people within the study, were going to be allowed to have AZT. But I said, "Like hell they are." So I sneaked looks in doctors' pathology books and wrote down three characteristic descriptions of the PCP bronchoscopy exam on my forged pathology report and took it to a doctor, who was suspicious, but fortunately agreeable. And that was submitted as evidence of my having had PCP, and within a week I was getting AZT.

I took AZT for 2 1/2 years. I actually tolerated it quite well but that was probably because I took it my own way. I calibrated my dosage of AZT down to 400 mg as early as 1987. Of course, only now in 1990, have they officially lowered the dose. Then, in the summer of 1989 I got ddI [didanosine (Videx)] through the underground and started that.

THE STRUGGLE TO KEEP WORKING

Q. *Is it hard to find the energy to keep going?*

A. Yes, it's nearly impossible sometimes. When I was lying on my couch, literally starving to death last fall—I was down to about 127 pounds—for me to get up and make the phone calls again, to find out more information, to know where I could get this object or that object which would be necessary for the infusion, etc., is what is called an "agon." It is a real struggle. That's why in this past year, with trying to get the contact here, and lining up doctors, and doing this and doing that in this ridiculous way, I was finally divorced from my identity, from my life's work, not from my job, because I didn't have a job. I had what I considered to be, at last, my life's work. Because I was forced to spend so much time, all of the time and energy I had left, negotiating my way around the medical system, I was finally cut off from my life. And now, my KS is out of control; I have MAI; I have CMV, and I have a horrible wasting syndrome which is barely under control. That is what my life has been reduced to. But if the medical system were responsive, I could still be doing a minimum amount of work. I certainly wouldn't be able to reinhabit my life to the fullest, but at least I would have some sense that my self was still there.

RAGE
Even though I spend every waking hour of the day working at this disease and working around the medical system, I'm not willing to throw in the towel no matter how hard it is emotionally, physically, and psychologically, because I know that this society, in general, has a death wish for Blacks and Hispanics and faggots. You're supposed to die. Anyone who tells you different is either a fool or a liar. They put the medical ring in your nose, and they lead you through a system which is a sham and a charade because they have nothing to say to you. It's as if you were an animal left behind the troop on the savannah, and you can just hear the jackals and the hyenas gathering around you. They make as much money as they possibly can by palming off on you the most technologically complex sort of medical intervention when it's already too late and you are supposed to die in the way that they want people to die. Because AIDS hit gay men first and then it hit the inner city Blacks and Hispanics, who were primarily drug users, this country unconsciously or consciously gets satisfaction out of seeing us die in a way that, according to them, we deserve. And I don't believe that having AIDS is demeaning in any way at all. I don't believe that having AIDS is ennobling in any way at all. Having AIDS is no different from having any other disease, but I refuse to lie down and die like a "faggot" should. And no one will ever convince me that they don't have a death wish for me because when Ronald Reagan didn't even know that AIDS existed for the first 5 years of his administration and nothing was done scientifically for so long in those initial years, there was only one reason. And if we are 5 years behind where we should be in medical research, it is solely because queers deserve to die from this. I listen to the news and I have to hear these bastards sitting there and saying that this is a self-inflicted disease. I probably got this virus in about 1976 or 1977. In order to have had symptoms by 1981, I definitely got this back in the 70s. Nobody even knew that this virus existed. But see, it's a choice. It's always a choice.

It's like being gay. Who in their right mind would choose to be gay in our culture? What 13-year-old kid with half a brain, knowing what happens, how difficult it is to be gay in our culture, will sit there and go, um, I'm going to be gay when I grow up. But of course, it's a choice because they have to be able to attribute volition to all of this. I'm so disgusted by that, so deeply repulsed by the ignorance and the fear and hatred of difference in this country, that that also is part of what drives me on, to just keep going and going and going. I mean, it doesn't give me any illusion that I'm going to survive this, because I'm not. Because no one has survived this.

NO ILLUSIONS

Q. *What has helped?*

A. I think the fact that I can think clearly about it, that I didn't lie to myself about it, that I didn't say, "Oh well, I'll be the one person, I'll be the star of my little musical here and at the end I'll come out and because I'm a good person, I won't die from this." I never lied to myself because I couldn't. Because I knew, you know, as many facts as I could know at the time. I knew what was at the end of the road, so it was a matter of being sober and clear-headed about it because I had seen too many people who had pretended everything would be all right because they were feeling well. You know, this always happens. People get out of the hospital, and they're really feeling good, and so they think that they're well. I was always just absolutely flabbergasted if not appalled by that attitude. I never let myself believe that everything was okay no matter how I was feeling. I think it was the force of my rational mind which had a lot to do with how soberly and deliberately I went about handling my situation.

FAMILY MATTERS

Q. *What was the most difficult aspect of all this for you at that time?*

A. My family. Thinking about my family. I'd never come out to my parents for a lot of reasons, but at least partly because I didn't even realize fully that I was gay until I was in my mid-twenties. I had been living away from my family since I was 18. They really hadn't been a part of my life for years and years. I didn't see any reason at all to approach them in a confessional mode, and I didn't see any reason to force them to prove that they loved me by accepting me because I was gay. I have lots of brothers and sisters, and as far as I know, my straight brothers and sisters have never gone to my parents to confess their heterosexuality or to explain it or anything. So I never felt compelled. When I was finally faced with this illness, it became a very big problem because now I couldn't tell them that I was sick without telling them that I was gay. I have a very deep resentment at having to tell them about my sexual life because if my older brother had cancer, he could tell my parents that he had cancer. They wouldn't then be confused and ashamed and fearful about his sexual life because he had cancer. So thinking about my family was very difficult. My family is extremely religious, and my parents are working class people who have only gotten through their lives by using religion as an explanation. By using the Catholic sort of world view to explain why their lives have been so difficult. They will only understand my illness through the filter of the Catholic world view.

Q. *Was it a while before you were actually able to tell them?*

A. I never told them, and I still haven't told them. Another reason why I decided not to tell them is that when I die, they're going to have the rest of their lives to suffer from this. They're going to wake up every morning with it on their minds and go to bed with it every night on their minds. They're going to have years to live with the fact that I died of this disease. I rarely go home. They're not wealthy people. There's nothing that they can do financially. My mother is nearly retired now. She's just 60, and my father is retired. I have seen no reason to add to their years of distress and fear and uncertainty and impotence by telling them every detail of this very difficult thing that I'm going through.

Q. *Are they aware of your having been ill?*

A. No. I think they may have noticed something only this past year when I went home at one point and I was looking rather sorry. Nothing was said then, of course. But when I came back to New York several weeks later, my Mom said that she was concerned that I looked too thin, etc., etc. But that's another aspect of it. My parents know that I'm gay. They just don't want to know that I'm gay.

Q. *What about your siblings? Is it the same story?*

A. It's hardly up to me to push their faces in it for any number of reasons. Knowing how hard my family will take it has been painful to me. My decision, the essence, the pith of my decision, has been that I can see no reason to drag them through the whole ugly thing. When the time comes, they're going to know, they're going to be at my bedside. I know that they love me. I know that I love them. And there is no reason to test that or draw out their pain and suffering a minute more than I have to. And when I'm on death's door, I'm sure that they'll be the first people there.

Q. *Were there other people that you chose to, or felt you had to, keep it from?*

A. No, just my family.

Q. *And you haven't actually gone out and told any family member?*

A. Well, I did. I told one brother who is gay. He's the other gay member of our litter. And S. is a sweetheart and whatnot, but S. can't bear too much reality. In the year since he's known that I've had AIDS, I've never gotten a phone call.

THE VALUE OF FRIENDSHIPS
Another aspect of this and the reason why I've been able to get to this point is the fact that, for some reason, although I've been unlucky in love, I have had a real talent for friendship over the years. If in this life I was blessed with one sort of social skill, it was making friends who were true, who are

devoted to me and love me. And if there was any question that my friends were really devoted to me and would stand by me every inch of the way, that was dispelled when I was in the hospital with toxoplasmosis. I can only think of two friends who simply were not able to handle it and have just rather dignifiedly slipped away. So that in terms of family, and telling my family, it wasn't as if I didn't have a family substitute—you know, people who were there with me day and night through all of the compound Q side effects. They do my shopping and clean my floors and do my dishes and pick up my laundry and do all of those things.

GOALS

Q. *What have you accomplished that you're particularly proud of?*

A. Well, I've stayed alive. Some of my literary translations are now considered standard. That happened well after I was first hospitalized. I continued to work a very long time, and I've managed to keep my friends, which is very difficult. Because when you're sick, it is very, very difficult to operate in the same world, with the same expectations, the same anything, as people who inhabit the land of the well. And mostly, if I haven't screamed at them, mostly I've managed to maintain some sort of dignity through it all, even though looking at healthy people is like walking around in a Plexiglas cylinder. You're deeply, deeply isolated from them, but there is no way a person who has what Susan Sontag calls full citizenship in the land of the ill could ever communicate to people who are not ill. And a lot of people lash out at people around them and blame them for the isolation that they feel in their illness. I struggle every day not to do that.

Q. *What about goals that you have now?*

A. I don't have any goals. My goal is not to have diarrhea tonight. My goal is to get food into my body today. I have contracts for projects that have languished on my desk for months and months now. I would love to do them, but I have radiation treatments three times a week. I have chemotherapy once a week. This week, I have three doctors' appointments and a dentist appointment. With severely depleted levels of energy, I think that that's about all I can be expected to do. Maybe that is the most difficult part of this whole thing—that when you become seriously ill with this or any other disease, the future is sloughed off and you become your past.

PHILOSOPHY

Q. *Early on, what did your doctors say about your prognosis? Were you led to believe that you would not survive as long as you have?*

A. Oh no. They would never say that. Even when M. called me from Mt. Sinai and said I'll give you a prescription for Bactrim, and I said to him, "Are you saying to me that I have AIDS?" "Oh no, not exactly. It depends on how you define it, etc., etc." I knew I wasn't going to get anything straight from him anyway, so my information about prognosis came from medical journals.

Q. *You seem to have taken a real active role in educating yourself and you've taken certain steps all on your own. Do you believe that the things you've done have helped keep you alive?*

A. Oh, yeah, yeah. Forging, smuggling, lying, cheating, everything short of extortion.

Q. *And some of the treatments that you have chosen and the medications themselves have....*

A. Well, I'd say that prophylaxis has been extremely important. Of course, that's something that no doctor ever thought of doing. The fact is that I take fluconazole for 10 days every month as prophylaxis against fungal infections. Of course that's going to keep me alive longer than people who don't receive prophylaxis against fungal infections. But I have fluconazole, which I got from England way back at the beginning of 1989. But I've had to do all of these practical things 100% on my own. And those things have absolutely kept me alive.

Q. *What are your thoughts about other more psychological approaches that people talk about to keep people going? You know, having a fighting spirit, the will to survive, the will to live, those kinds of things. Where do you stand on that?*

A. Well, I'm something of a snob about this. What I depend on is just trying to be rational and sober and as realistic as I possibly can about the whole thing. I have no illusions that I'm not going to die of AIDS. But, what I have a certain amount of control over is the manner in which I die of AIDS. I mean, anybody can think anything they want. If something helps, fine. I have absolutely no right to make a judgement about what anybody does in terms of emotional or psychological strategies to get them through. Personally, I don't like fantasies or the silliness.

PLANNING THE END: WHEN ENOUGH IS ENOUGH

Q. *Do you ever feel like it's not worth it? Do you feel like giving up?*

A. Yeah, a lot, particularly since I started wasting and started having the intestinal things and the DHPG failed. And then the gastroenterologist tells me, "Well, there's really nothing we can do about this because we don't know anything about it." You know, when someone tells you that and you're spending your entire day passing brown flux on the stool and you look like hell, you want to die. And when the KS lesions on my face just out-number the number of times that I can go and have radiation, yeah, I just want to say, "Fuck it."

And the fact is that I have made provisions to be able to do just that when I so choose. Because I have six bags of very strong heroin, which I've had for quite a while now. I know how to put them into solution and....

Q. *You said "quite a while." When did you first....*

A. Well, I've been trying to get Seconal or Nembutal for years, from the very beginning, actually. But of course, nobody could get it, you know. No medical professional could ever write a prescription in triplicate like that. I went to the underground for ddI; I went to the underground for compound Q; I finally turned to forgery to get the AZT; and I went to the streets to get the heroin.

Q. *So you've got the heroin and you're clear about that.*

A. Yes, I know how to put it into solution and there's no problem at all. All I need is the heplock in my arm, and that's easy enough.

Q. *When would you do that? What would it take? How would you know the time had come?*

A. When the signs of the disease on me are so strong that I no longer recognize myself in the mirror as anything but the undead version of the person that I was. That psychological aspect—when I actually feel as if there is no more left of me in my physical body—that's part of it. There's also the simple suffering—when I get too skinny, when I have too many perianal CMV lesions, when I can't swallow, when I suffocate from my throat being closed by thrush or something. Then there's just the pure physical thing. I don't think there's anything ennobling about lying there and drawing it out further and further. I mean, in my mind, there is a real problem in the way that science and medicine have been confused. And I don't care about what any self-righteous doctor says about doing everything he can until the end. That is science and I need medicine. The distinction is clear in my mind. If they want to drag me to a hospital, intubate me, and put me on a respirator—that is just making money. Anyone who tells you different is a fool or a liar. It is not for the patient. It is for their own sense of heroic capacity as doctors. Intervention with all of this technology is a symptom of a hideous hubris that permeates the medical profession in this country.

Q. *Do you feel you have control over whether or not this happens to you?*

A. Yeah, I've decided twice already not to go to the hospital when others were at me to go. I mean, I've scrambled and struggled and fought and done everything in my capacity to be in control of this as much as possible. At the end, I'm not just going to lie back and let those predators move in on me.

Q. *Do you find yourself feeling discouraged? Are you sad, even depressed? Do you feel hopeless?*

A. Yeah. I'd say that I'm depressed all the time. I have a cosmic existential sadness that could never, ever be totally resolved, even if I were to wake up tomorrow completely healthy. This may be my own form of hubris or pride or whatever, but the fact is that I was on the verge of a terrific life. I was a workingman's son who made it through the Ivy League on sheer grit and hard work, who opted out of the official system to pursue something that I loved: literature and language. I was trying to move my grain of culture up the beach of civilization. I believed in it. I did everything that I had to do to really make something of it, and then the rug was pulled out from under me. How could you not feel sad about that?

Q. *What kinds of things help when you are feeling discouraged?*

A. Nothing. If I'm feeling discouraged, there is nothing that can be done about it. I break things, I throw things, I curse at strangers. Sometimes I yell at friends.

Q. *And at those times, how do your friends react?*

A. They're mostly amazingly understanding. Having people around always helps. When I'm feeling so discouraged that I can't even go and make my own dinner, it helps if there's someone in the kitchen cooking for me. But the depth of the despair gnaws away at you. After the uncertainty and fear and physical difficulties, this rodent has eaten all the way through my heart and you can't ask it to cough it up. After all, I've been aware that something's wrong for 9 years.

Q. *Do you find yourself thinking about death a lot?*

A. Yes. I think about it all the time.

Q. *All the time?*

A. All the time because I'm going to die from this. And because all I would have to do to die from this is just to say "uncle." That's all I have to do.

Q. *What are your views on life and death? What are your views about what happens when someone dies?*

A. I believe that when you're dead, you're probably dead…period. Hopefully you have done something here in the face of all the meaninglessness, in the face of the nothingness, in the face of what might actually be a cosmic joke, that you stood your ground and held yourself to a level of activity that could in some way dignify your having lived. That's about it.

Q. *You recently described your mood as depressed.*

A. I would say I'm depressed all the time, yes. But more than depressed, I'm enraged. My dominant emotion is rage. I want to kill people. I want to smash things. I want to give the finger to God, that kind of stuff. I break things at home. I'm mostly angry from sheer frustration at being denied my life. That's what it is. I'm angry because I'm lost to my life, and I'm frustrated, and I want it back. But I know that the chances are virtually nil that I will get it back, which makes me even more angry. And if I start thinking about it, then I get depressed. But mostly I would like to kill other people rather than myself. Medical people mostly.

Q. *Are you able to enjoy things the way you used to be able to?*

A. No, not at all. Not at all. Barely a vestige. Joy is not part of my life. The things that gave me the most pleasure don't give me joy.

EPILOGUE

Bill died 3 months after this interview, in early summer. In his last winter, he spent Christmas, Valentine's Day, St. Patrick's Day, Easter, and Passover in the hospital. Throughout, he was surrounded by friends. According to one friend, also very ill and also in the hospital with him on those holidays, his friends were loyal to the end, "even though he was unbearable to be with." On Easter, for example, "Fifteen or 20 of his friends came in and hand-dyed Easter eggs in the traditional Russian way. They hand painted them with tiny brushes and gave them away to everyone in the hospital. He was, paradoxically, loved by many, many people. Just cherished by so many, and his memorial service was heartbreaking and about 3 hours long because everybody wanted to speak."

Bill meets all the criteria of a "good" patient, as defined by both physicians and patients. He was willing to take charge of his life and his medical care. He was informed; he was honest with his doctors; he was observant about symptomatic changes; and he persisted in his professional activities for the first 6 years of his illness. But Bill was also an impossible patient in many respects. He trusted nobody, refused to work in a partnership regarding his medical management, and was difficult and irascible not only with professionals but also with his friends.

Bill's point of view is not unique. If it were, this story would not be informative. He expresses the fears and frustrations that many people with AIDS feel at one time or another, especially as they enter a period of decline. His loathing for the medical profession, his refusal or inability to find a physician he could work with and trust, his apparent detachment from others with AIDS, are extreme examples of the periods of fear and anger at both man and God that many PWAs experience and move beyond.

Bill's story represents a more consistent aversion toward the medical establishment than is usually expressed. Most people tend to fluctuate: something changes about their treatment or response, and they get back into the medical system. Most people find a way to make compromises, to go on with life, to adapt somehow, to find some sources of pleasure in their day, to make something a source of happiness. And, as we will discuss later, most people with AIDS have some sense of hope, even about death. When interviewed, Bill was more despairing and angry than most, yet he struggled in his own way to the very end.

2

THE GOOD HIV PATIENT: PHYSICIAN PERSPECTIVES

COMMENT

People who cope well with HIV illness also tend to cope well with life in general, adapting and growing in response to difficult challenges. It often appears that HIV acts as a magnifying lens, enlarging personality characteristics, both positive and negative. In many respects, the effective HIV-positive patient is simply an effective human being. Nevertheless, a variety of useful skills and behaviors that can enhance care and potentially prolong survival can be learned. From the physician's perspective these patient skills include learning how to participate in medical care, being informed, being honest, and being vigilant. Being a long-term AIDS survivor is partly a biologic phenomenon, influenced by treatment; partly emotional, spiritual, and psychological, influenced by attitude; and partly a matter of focusing on survival as a task that involves skill and competency. Patients can, to a certain extent, shape their experiences by learning how to facilitate their own care.

While good medical care is often central to long-term survival, it is not sufficient: The patient must actively participate in his or her own care as well. "Good" patients, from the physician's perspective, take charge of their own situations, assuming responsibility for their own health and well-being. Such behavior requires acknowledging that HIV illness tends to be progressive, that symptoms and infections are likely to occur despite months or years of extended good health, and that, at some point, life may change dramatically.

Taking charge of one's health and planning ahead is difficult. First, when is it appropriate to start thinking about the possibility of illness? When should one begin to make contingency plans in case health changes? Second, taking responsibility entails an acknowledgement of potential illness and a foreshortened life. Third, there are potentially negative ramifications to "taking charge" and thus defining oneself as a patient, ranging from a possible rebuff by friends and family to undesirable consequences at work or in living arrangements. Furthermore, planning usually implies an ability to anticipate, with at least some accuracy, the timing and nature of future events. Since one of the hallmarks of HIV illness is unpredictability, planning involves a great deal of uncertainty. Nevertheless, the consequences of failing to do so become increasingly evident as illness becomes progressive.

A surprising number of otherwise competent and effective people avoid taking responsibility for their health and their futures. A vivid description of the perils of this neglect was offered by a highly respected AIDS physician:

> One of the things I find most frustrating is patients not planning for change in their status, in terms of their jobs, in terms of their insurance, and in terms of the problems it gives their doctors, their families and other people around them. I'd say, "Look, you have to deal with the fact that you have this problem and there are a lot of signs that the disease is progressing. You can't pretend this is not happening, unless this is your *conscious choice.* You know you are not in a relationship; you own an apartment, and you co-own a beach house. You have a responsible job, and your coworkers don't know that you're sick or anything. And you're not out to your family in Iowa that you're gay. Your T cells are 50, and although you look fine, what's the scenario here? Do you want to be the person at the health club, who has a seizure and crashes into the mirrored wall and then ends up in the emergency room? When my business card is found on you, the hospital will call me, asking, who are you, what's your medical history. Who is going to give permission for the lumbar puncture?" I'd ask the patient, "Is that how you want your mother in Iowa, who is 73 years old, to find out that you're gay and have a terminal disease? When you're already in a coma? Is this what you want? Because if that's what you want, fine. As long as I know that's how you want it to be. Even though I can't imagine that, we'll have to play it out. But if that's not the way you want it, then you really have to take charge and think about some issues and make some arrangements now."

By confronting the patient in this way, the physician focuses on the need to accept responsibility, to anticipate, and to be prepared for change, even by people at risk who have not been seriously ill. Because of the uncertainties that characterize HIV disease, the key is not to have a single plan but to develop contingencies.

HELPFUL BEHAVIORS

When physicians talk about "assuming responsibility for one's health," they generally mean that patients should engage in certain helpful behaviors. These include taking an active part in one's medical care, being informed, being honest with the physician, and being vigilant about one's health (observing and reporting). A fifth quality, while not specifically a doctor-patient interaction, also appears common among effective patients, namely, the willingness to maintain a "normal" life as long as health permits. Efforts to keep going appear to influence physicians' perceptions and appraisals of patients.

THE "GOOD" HIV PATIENT

- Takes responsibility for and charge of his or her health
- Acknowledges that HIV illness is usually progressive and makes plans based on a variety of contingencies
- Is informed about the natural history of HIV disease and keeps current about changing treatment recommendations
- Observes and reports symptoms to the physician promptly
- Considers the physician a trustworthy working partner with whom he or she is honest and open
- Complies with agreed on treatment regimens
- Practices a healthy lifestyle
- Maintains as normal a life as possible for as long as possible
- Has a positive attitude toward the value of life and personal worth
- Keeps track of prescriptions and understands their purpose
- Utilizes medical appointments efficiently by preparing a list of concerns and questions
- Expresses appreciation on occasion to a physician who is caring and concerned
- Accepts, and seeks, help when necessary
- Devotes sufficient time to medical care
- Has realistic expectations, but continues to set and work toward goals

---

Active Participation in Medical Care

Physicians emphasize the importance of patient cooperation, such as taking medications as prescribed, reporting all symptoms, and being honest. From the physician's perspective, "The good patient is the one who takes care of his body, who takes the medications that he has agreed to take. He calls when he's sick; he reads and learns about his condition, asks questions, challenges me. A good patient is usually a put-together person in general; they are few and far between."

One physician indicated, "I like patients to be organized so that when they come to see me they can tell me what their problems are and maybe even give me a list. I hate it when almost as they're leaving, they say, 'Oh, by the way, I had a fever of 110 last week. Do you think that's significant?'"

Another physician, who had not encountered many patients who met his expectations, noted that HIV disease is a good model for American health care in general:

> In terms of health care, we are guilty as a society of irresponsibility. We want the best of everything, but we don't want to have to take responsibility. We simply don't want to be held accountable for having to do anything. That's a sweeping generalization, but I'm amazed at patients who are too willing to give in, to give up control. Under other circumstances these same people wouldn't think of allowing their businesses to go unsupervised, for example. And yet these very individuals can be remarkably irresponsible in terms of their own medical care. I'm not talking about people who are so sick that they are unable. I'm referring to patients in relatively good shape who never know if they have refills or even what medicines they're taking. A lot of people will tell you stuff like, "Well I know you said from where my counts are at that I have to go to the eye doctor every 6 months, but I sort of lost track."
>
> I want to say to these patients, "You have a problem whether you want it or not, and you have to take charge of it the same way you take charge of your life in other areas. If I lost track of the fact that you're on AZT and hadn't watched your hemoglobin over the last 6 months until it reached a critical level, that would be inexcusable! Well, why is your behavior any more excusable?" We're at a point now where the delivery of medical care is very sophisticated, but it's got to be a two-way street.

Some may say that this physician sounds angry and demands a great deal from his patients, expecting a degree of responsibility that is unrealistic for some patients. Perhaps he is. Nevertheless, his expectations might be said to represent the ideal or "gold standard" of behaviors that promote optimal health and contribute to long-term survival for all people living with HIV illness. The degree to which patients can approximate a high level of responsibility in partnership with their physicians will determine how close they come to ideal behavior.

Being Informed

Effective management of HIV disease requires that the patient be informed about the natural history of the infection, its manifestations, and various treatment options and strategies. Being informed can be a difficult, time consuming, and ongoing endeavor. Moreover, treatment recommendations are constantly being altered as experts interpret findings and implications of new studies and as new medications become available. What may have been considered standard treatment 4 months ago may not be so clear-cut today.

Some patients seem to feel, "If I have little time left, I surely don't want to spend it dealing with textbooks and treatment newsletters. That's the doctor's job. Let the doctor keep track of it all. It just uses up my time and makes me nervous." Nevertheless, experienced AIDS specialists believe that patients should try to gain an understanding of the entire picture, of the course of illness, and of its natural history. "It really makes my life easier," one physician explained, "when you don't have to start from ground zero." The patient needs to know what problems to anticipate and how to identify symptoms when they occur. Equally important is an understanding of what problems are highly unlikely.

The good patient is aware of "what his treatment regimen is, where he is, and where he's going." If a treatment plan makes sense to the patient, he is more likely to cooperate with it. A naive or ill-informed patient can be frustrating for the physician. "I actually resent someone who comes in and doesn't know anything. As obnoxious as it can be, as much as I sometimes hate what patients read—because they come in with these new theories or questions about treatments they've heard of—the worst thing is ignorance. I prefer to treat people who are basically informed, rational, realistic, and who participate."

Awareness of probable outcome is also important in being an effective patient, particularly in the setting of significant illness. Some physicians observed: "Patients who cope better with AIDS are those who have seen the disease in the community. They understand what it is. They've lived with it, they know what the likely outcome is." Another said, "The good patient knows that our current treatments are not cures."

Challenging the Physician

Physicians vary in their willingness to be challenged by patients who come to them with their own ideas. Some specialists actively prefer this kind of patient: "In my practice, a good patient, one whom I would consider likely to survive longer, is one who is knowledgeable, asks questions, makes proposals himself or herself, and questions what I have to say. The inquiring patient brings useful suggestions to the physician, reads newsletters, and is aware of the changing field. Such an individual might be a nuisance but would be a good patient and I like that." Others prefer a slightly less "in-your-face" attitude from patients.

Being Honest with the Physician

A third characteristic of helpful behavior is honesty about treatment adherence. Treatment regimens may appear unnecessary in early-stage disease and are often arduous, difficult, and unpleasant in late-stage illness. Nonadherence to prescribed treatment appears to be an important issue for physicians: "I like patients to be honest and tell me they disagree with my advice," one physician said. "I want to know if they don't want to take the medication or the test. I don't think deceiving the physician to make him or her happy is a very good thing, and I tell patients up front that I really want them to be honest." Physicians need to know if the patient decides to stop taking a medication: "Tell me, ask me questions. I want to hear the reason why things didn't work out."

Since good physicians recognize the potential for healing, if not cure, of "supplemental" treatments, such as acupuncture, chiropractic care, or Chinese herbs, patients who seek such approaches should be honest about them. Physicians usually recognize psychological benefit, as well as the possible physical benefit, of such therapies. Most believe very strongly, however, that such therapies should not be used exclusively, to replace more standard and effective treatments. Patients should talk openly with their physicians about incorporating supplemental treatments into their overall care. Another irritating and potentially dangerous form of dishonesty that clearly stands in the way of optimal medical care is failure to tell a physician that one has already consulted with another specialist and is on medication.

Healthy Vigilance: Observing and Reporting

The fourth behavior that good patients exhibit is accurate and timely observation and reporting of new symptoms or changes in health status: "I think that patients are my first line of defense against the illness by being my eyes and ears. They have to know what to look for and what to bring to my attention. The worst scenario for an AIDS doctor is the patient who comes in on death's doorstep because he had the flu that wouldn't go away, lost 30 pounds, can't breathe, and never called. So it's helpful when patients come to us early with significant symptoms."

The effective patient is one who is in tune with his or her own body. The patient's report: "'Something's going on. I don't know exactly what it is, but I don't feel as well this month as last month' is just as important as the results of an abnormal blood study."

Vigilance Versus Hypochondriasis

Recognizing the difference between appropriate vigilance and hypochondriasis is a more complicated issue than physicians sometimes acknowledge. Patients often don't know when to call the physician and seldom are given specific guidelines by the doctor. How does one distinguish a flu from *Pneumocystis carinii* pneumonia (PCP) or sore throat from possible thrush? How many days does one wait with a fever or a cough before calling? What about pain? When does one decide that a new medication isn't working? Many patients are so apprehensive about "crying wolf" that they may suffer considerable distress before notifying their doctors. Others find that telephone calls aren't returned for many hours or even days and are then discouraged from subsequent efforts.

Other patients, however, think nothing of calling the doctor late at night about a symptom, such as a rash, that they noticed during the day. And some would like to obtain advice and counsel by phone so they don't have to deal with the inconvenience or cost of an office visit.

This particular skill—health vigilance—requires that physicians educate their patients and demonstrate concern by being responsive and returning phone calls. Physicians vary in their expectations about when patients should call, and they vary in their willingness or ability to return calls promptly. This often becomes an important issue for negotiation between doctor and patient.

GENERAL ADVICE: SEEK CARE EARLY

A wise patient offered the following good advice: "I call my physician when something new is happening to my body, something that I haven't had before, that I don't understand, that's persistent or keeps recurring. I listen to my body very carefully. I don't call when I think it's something that I've had before, that I'm familiar with and can handle."

Patients should report new symptoms, particularly if they persist for more than 48 hours, to their doctors. When in doubt, it is generally better to err on the side of being too cautious than to neglect potentially significant changes. In many cases, the patient can be reassured that "it's nothing to worry about." A brief discussion with the physician can be extremely helpful in reducing anxiety.

Patients who call repeatedly with insignificant concerns might be appropriately counseled about when and why to contact the physician. A printed list of potentially serious symptoms, for example, may help such patients decide when to seek medical advice. An effective doctor-patient relationship, worked out relatively early in the course of illness, will benefit both parties.

Besides the fear of being labeled a hypochondriac, many patients are reluctant to report new symptoms because these may indicate a serious problem. They may hope that the new symptoms will disappear within a few days. Nobody who has been asymptomatic with HIV infection wants to be confronted with a diagnosis of an illness that may reclassify him as having AIDS. Likewise, the patient who has already weathered one opportunistic infection doesn't want to find out that another one has arisen. Nevertheless, early intervention in a treatable illness may be life-saving; it may also avert hospitalization, result in a shorter treatment period, and prevent discomfort, weight loss, and further complications.

Notifying the physician of new symptoms requires effort and specific skills. It may be difficult to get through to the doctor, to know what type of message to leave, or how to describe the problem clearly and succinctly. And, waiting to hear from the physician can be anxiety provoking. It is usually helpful if another doctor in the office, or a nurse, or physician assistant, is available to offer a preliminary response and to convey the patient's concern to the physician.

MAINTAINING A NORMAL LIFE

The effective patient continues to live as normal a life as possible, rather than leaping prematurely into the role of illness. Even with a CD4 count of 50, he or she is still interested in going to work or engaging in some meaningful activity.

Living a normal life knowing that one is HIV-positive can be a great challenge. Meeting that challenge involves all aspects of life: outlook and attitude, social ties, occupational activity, and indeed, one's very identity. The extent to which outlook remains largely optimistic, that ties with others are sustained or even bolstered, that accomplishment in one's work continues to bring gratification, and that one maintains a core identity will determine how effective that person is likely to be as a successful partner in his or her own medical management.

Patients who do well are not consumed by their diagnosis and continue to work when capable, maintain relationships, and make plans for the future. Having plans and looking forward to them is perhaps more important than whether or not they can actually be carried out. While it may be that one needs to feel physically well to remain active, there appears to be a relationship between activity level, future outlook, health status, and survival.

Social Relationships

Apart from the inherent pleasure of connections to other people, having social ties can influence physical health and survival. "I've always felt," commented a physician, "for cancer patients or in any other disease, that once people feel abandoned and unwanted, or that nobody cares, they usually give up. And when people give up on themselves, they die very fast." Friends can offer advice, arrange medical care, and generally help with concrete needs and services. One physician noticed, "People who have lots of support do better. That's friends and family and insurance and employers and doctors. In every aspect of their lives, they do better. A person who is connected to the world is going to get a lot more assistance, such as reminders to keep appointments or help in getting medications filled, which leads to adherence. These are major determinants."

Physicians generally understand that companionship contributes to good health and being an effective patient: "A good AIDS patient is someone who will not allow himself to be isolated but who will turn to friends for support. If I see a patient who works long hours, lives alone, and never goes out, I encourage that patient to go to support groups, because having people to talk to, share, and go through difficult times with, makes a big difference."

A patient who is isolated can also present management difficulties:

> The highest risk patients are those who live alone. If they become incontinent, bed-bound, or mentally impaired, it's very difficult to maintain them at home. When someone with no white cells is hospitalized, there's a flag that identifies him as a high risk for infection. Social services should have a flag for AIDS patients who live alone as the single highest risk group.

Living alone while physically still able to manage independently may not in itself be a significant risk. Individuals with good friends and/or sympathetic family members who visit and who would be available to help out at times of acute illness don't generally represent a problem, especially if insurance permits arrangements for home attendants.

Another pattern of social isolation is sometimes seen in the surviving member of couples who are both ill. After the death of one, the other may lose interest in the struggle to survive, may be unwilling to form new attachments, and may even go so far as to discourage friends and family members from staying involved in his or her welfare and daily life.

The same concern is expressed about parents who are HIV-positive and lose one or more children to the disease. Typically, parents may have neglected themselves in the struggle to care for a child. When a parent loses a child to AIDS, the grief can be overwhelming and may lead to depression and a desire to "give up." Like the individual who has lost a spouse or lover, a person surviving a child's death is especially vulnerable to losing interest in and withdrawing from the world. Often, however, the needs and demands of other children or family members will keep a surviving parent going. As one advocate for women with AIDS said, "The demands on the women I see are so overwhelming, they sometimes don't even have time to grieve the loss of a child, unless it is their only child. Others in the family don't stop needing, so she keeps on doing for others." Having others that need or are dependent on the patient may be, in part, a protective factor when surviving a significant and devastating loss. More generally, the presence of spouses, lovers, family, companions, and confidantes seems to contribute significantly to quality of life, and perhaps, to health, as well. As one physician observed, "AIDS is not a good disease to have alone."

Work

Physicians generally feel that continuing to work keeps people in the mainstream of life as long as they have the energy and mental acuity to do so. One physician actually started an organization that provides flexible work opportunities for people with AIDS, whose mission "is to keep people normal." The general belief is that, other things being equal, people are better off working. "I encourage everybody to work. If people have a plan for what they'll do if they're not working, then I say go ahead—sometimes it's appropriate. Most of my patients, however, thrive on work."

The goal is to have some focus other than illness: "People who do well are those who don't let the disease take over their lives. It seems that work matters. I really discourage my patients from stopping work unless I feel they can't handle it. He's just going to sit home all day and obsess over the disease." Regarding the effects of work-related stress, one physician stated, "If people are able to work, like their work, and are involved in it, that's good stress. Even if it's high stress, it isn't a drawback. I encourage patients to continue working unless they have really awful jobs."

There are circumstances in which physicians do question the wisdom of continuing to work. Some occupations, for example, can pose risks to health. Others may be too physically demanding. In general, however, patients are encouraged to work as long as they can, particularly if they can modify the demands of the job as their health changes.

Identity

Occasionally, some patients become so involved with being a person with AIDS (PWA) that it becomes their central identity. As one physician explained, "There are patients who keep going to AIDS conferences and scan every poster looking for the cure. That's unreasonable. They're desperate. AIDS has so overwhelmed their lives that there is nothing left. They do not enjoy life at all. They're miserable." This behavior is as maladaptive as is its opposite: denial. If life has been reasonably gratifying, the patient who remains the person he used to be before diagnosis is likely to fare better.

THE DIFFICULT PATIENT

Certain patients are difficult to work with. The socially isolated, as previously mentioned, can present problems. The narcissistic person often makes unreasonable demands and can also be quite difficult. A central feature of this type is failure to recognize the professional nature of the doctor-patient relationship.

> Most people are reasonable, but some think you should be at their beck and call, that they can call you 24 hours a day. It's two o'clock in the morning, and they just got home from a bar and were thinking about something. They were wondering what you thought about it. You want to just put a shotgun to that person's head. That's an unreasonable patient.

Difficult patients are encountered in all areas of medicine. They may be passive about their treatment, fail to report significant health changes, fail to keep track of their regimens, neglect to mention self-initiated changes in medications, and, in general, fail to treat the physician as a respected working partner. Some have grating personalities, while others have absolutely no personal or social resources, depending exclusively on the medical team. These patients are fairly easy to identify and to manage; there is, however, another type of patient, fortunately uncommon, who evokes positive dread in most physicians.

A now famous paper that appeared in *The New England Journal of Medicine* was entitled "Taking Care of the Hateful Patient" (Groves, 1978). The author noted, "Emotional reactions to patients cannot simply be wished away, nor is it good medicine to pretend that they do not exist" (p 883). Four "stereotypes" are delineated, all characterized by various manifestations of dependency. The *clinger* evokes aversion; *demanders* evoke a wish to counterattack; *help-rejecters* evoke depression; and *self-destructive deniers* evoke feelings of malice. The ability to recognize such patients may be a successful tool used by doctors and other caregivers to guide treatment plans and goals.

The Dependent Clinger

"Clingers escalate from mild requests for reassurance to repeated, perfervid, incarcerating cries for explanation, affection, analgesics, sedatives, and all forms of attention imaginable. They are naive about their effect on the physician, and they are overt in their neediness. What is common to them is their self-perception of bottomless need and their perception of the physician as inexhaustible. Such dependency may eventually lead to a sense of weary aversion toward the patient" (Groves, 1978, p 884).

Entitled Demanders

Demanders, like clingers, exhibit profound neediness. However, to achieve their goals, they use intimidation, devaluation, and guilt-induction. "They buttress their hold on the doctor by threatening punishment. The patient is unaware of the deep dependency that underlies these attacks on the doctor. The physician, in turn, does not recognize that the hostility is born of a terror of abandonment. Moreover, such patients often exude a repulsive sense of innate deservedness as if they were far superior to the physician"(Groves, 1978, p 885).

Manipulative Help-Rejecters

These patients "appear to feel that no regimen will help. Appearing almost smugly satisfied, they return again and again to the office or clinic to report that, once again, the regimen did not work. When one of their symptoms is relieved, another mysteriously appears to take its place. Apparently, what is sought is not relief of symptoms. What is sought is an undivorceable marriage to an inexhaustible caregiver"(Groves, 1978, p 885).

Self-Destructive Deniers

Not all deniers are self-destructive. An example of one who is would be the patient with esophageal varices and hepatic failure who continues to drink. These patients "appear to find their main pleasure in defeating the physician's attempts to preserve their lives. They may represent a chronic form of suicidal behavior; often they let themselves die"(Groves, 1978, p 886).

While these types of patients may afflict any practice, they probably appear less often in the offices of HIV specialists than elsewhere. The sense of urgency and limited time imposed by the nature of the disease tend to force patients to "get real." Nevertheless, HIV infection doesn't cause personality changes, and the "hateful patient" may make an appearance.

REFERENCE

Groves JE. Taking care of the hateful patient. *The New England Journal of Medicine.* 1978;298:883–887.

3

THE GOOD HIV PATIENT: PATIENT PERSPECTIVES

COMMENT
Talking to people with AIDS about what constitutes an effective patient and the factors that contribute to long-term survival elicits more complex responses than posing the same questions to physicians. Patients describe adaptive behaviors at different stages of illness rather than a global set of attributes. Patients also place a greater emphasis on the role of attitude and other "inner resources" than do physicians. What patients recognize is that having a positive attitude appears to be a prerequisite to engaging in specific behaviors that are likely to contribute to long-term survival. Without a positive attitude there is a greater tendency to passivity, to let the disease "run its course." Three broad stages of the disease, which dictate overlapping as well as specific strategies and resources have been observed.

ASYMPTOMATIC STAGE
The patient's first major task after learning that he or she is HIV positive is self-education. Perhaps most important, the person has to learn what resources are available for information and assistance. Ancillary issues, such as occupational, legal, insurance, and living situations, must also be considered. At this stage, a willingness and ability to take charge, to become informed, and to recognize the importance of a good doctor-patient relationship are the predominant characteristics of the "good" patient.

An additional psychological task is to avoid conceiving of the diagnosis as a death sentence, to remain hopeful, and to maintain normalcy in day-to-day functioning. For middle-class men and women, there is likely to be an extended period characterized by relatively good health in the absence of symptoms, or with only transient and episodic events. Among the poor and less educated, this asymptomatic phase of HIV infection is often not known because many first discover their serostatus during an emergency hospitalization for an acute opportunistic infection.

During this asymptomatic phase, self-education should include the natural history of HIV illness as it is currently understood, the indices of immune status and general health, options to be considered for prophylactic treatments, and physical changes that must be reported. At the outset, the newly identified HIV-positive person needs to carefully select a physician whom he or she considers to be encouraging and positive as well as knowledgeable and experienced. The patient must "first feel entitled to ask questions and say to him or herself, 'I have to think carefully about this.' You must talk to people; start going to groups and developing a sense of where you fit. You must determine what feels right for you and communicate that to your doctor."

Here is the story of a woman, an effective or "good" patient, who struggled against numerous obstacles to obtain the best medical care available:

> When I first went for care, I found out there was an infectious disease clinic. The staff told me that I had to wait until I got sicker before I could be seen in that clinic. But I wanted to see the doctors who were seeing people who had full-blown AIDS because they had a lot of information. I figured they might be able to help me before I got to that stage. I couldn't see why you had to wait until you were really sick to be in this clinic.
>
> A friend of mine said that she had the best doctor who knew all about AIDS. As soon as I heard that I started to go to that clinic. I went to three appointments and all three times I saw different providers, not all of whom were doctors. I wanted firsthand care from a physician. My friend told me that she was seeing a doctor there who worked at that clinic only one day of the week. So I went to his office, and I asked to see him separately. I told him that I wanted 5 minutes of his time. He agreed to see me even though he was very busy. I sat down and told him who I was and that I was HIV-positive, and I had heard he was the best. I explained that when I was on drugs I had looked for the best drugs and now that I had HIV, this is a true story, I was looking for the best HIV doctor, because it's the way I do things. I told him that I wanted him to be my doctor. He laughed and he said, "I would be glad to be your doctor."

Her story does not end there because she realized that she needed to remain actively involved as a partner in her own care.

> Well, I became his patient; I went to the clinic on his days only; and I only saw him. There were times when he was very busy, and I would say, "No, I want to see him." Somehow I knew that it was important to see the same provider all the time who would know about my medical condition, about what was going on with me, and would know me personally. I wanted to establish a relationship, so that's how I made sure I saw the same person all the time. Sometimes I was in the clinic for 6 hours, literally, but this pushy bitch is alive after 8 1/2 years and doing well.

SYMPTOMATIC STAGE

Once laboratory measures indicate significant immunosuppression, when constitutional symptoms develop, or an episodic infection occurs, patients need to take a new approach to interactions with their doctors. At this stage, honesty about adherence to the agreed on treatment plan and careful observation and reporting of health changes become crucial.

Maintaining Normalcy

It is during these first two stages of HIV disease that "maintaining normalcy" at work and in social relationships becomes most salient. Some people, at times encouraged by their physicians, leave work and go on disability because of anticipated concern about work-related stress, which could be detrimental to their health. They may then remain essentially healthy for months or years, and in the future may come to regret this "wasted" time. This is a theme recurrently cited by long-term survivors when considering what they would have done differently in the time since their diagnosis: "After I was diagnosed with PCP [*Pneumocystis carinii* pneumonia], I stopped what I was doing and rented a house in Connecticut, thinking 'This is the last house I'll see.' It was by a lake, and it was very pretty, and I went out there and just laid back and waited to die. But, it didn't happen. Now I see I wasted 2 years waiting for the disease to strike, so I stopped waiting to die by the lake and came back and got on with my life."

CHRONIC ILLNESS

Contrary to popular belief, the lives of people who are HIV-positive are not substantially altered by illness on a day-to-day basis. If they do develop symptoms or infections, these often are episodic and limited, with return to a baseline level of health and functioning being common. Eventually, however, a later stage may be reached where illness becomes the predominant factor of life. Today, people live longer after diagnosis of an AIDS-defining condition, and additional effective prophylaxis and treatment of the episodic opportunistic infections like PCP and toxoplasmosis are being developed. Consequently, the first serious chronic illness experienced by persons with AIDS (PWAs) may be a condition like cytomegalovirus (CMV). More people are living longer and entering this phase. It is at this juncture that additional personality attributes and specific abilities appear necessary to sustain a satisfying life and promote survival.

People who have lived for extended periods with significant and chronic illness ultimately relinquish their former lives and devote their attention to survival. At this point, the effective patient must let AIDS-related medical regimens and activities dominate the day, nearly every day, in effect making AIDS their central "job." Patients must stay abreast of new treatment options when standard treatments are no longer effective; maintain confidence in their physicians; be able to accept help from others (either professionals or friends/family); and have faith that life is worth fighting for.

Fighting Late-Stage Disease: A Case Study

Many of these themes were articulated by a young man who had his first opportunistic infection 5 years earlier and who had been receiving daily I.V.

therapy for CMV for the past 2 years. At the time of the interview, neither ganciclovir (Cytovene) nor foscarnet (Foscavir) were controlling his CMV retinitis or colitis; he was losing his vision; he had severe gastrointestinal problems, including weight loss and chronic diarrhea; and he was experiencing what was probably CMV-induced reticulopathy causing problems with balance. He spent over 3 hours a day receiving infusions for CMV and recently had chosen to discontinue I.V. feeding, which required another 12 hours a day, because "it was taking too high a price out of my life." This is his analysis of the effective patient:

> To be really effective as a patient, AIDS has to be your central agenda, your new career. I suspect a lot of PWAs die prematurely because they just can't or won't give the disease the attention it requires for survival. That's probably not talked about much, but feeling myself lose the energy needed to go through my whole regimen every day makes me realize how many other people must have the same experience. Finally they just give up taking *all* the treatments and taking *all* the pills. It's all so medical and it's all so time-consuming. If I were undergoing experimental treatments, as well as exploring new options and doing massage and yoga, it would be a 12-hour day. I can't bring myself to do all that. That's probably the gold standard patient. I'm more of a reluctant one. As the time required for all the I.V. infusions gets longer, I get worse and worse at it. I so resent the time it takes out of my day, where I can be a normal person. I think the ability to function as an effective patient is really a stamina and energy issue.
>
> Another quality of a good patient, unfortunately, is the ability to allow other people to take over your life. You have to be able to withstand the embarrassment of becoming dependent on other people, which can be very humiliating. You have to subordinate your ego and not worry any more about being independent. I think a lot of people can't take that.
>
> I've been dizzy for about 2 months to the point where it's hard to walk on the street, and I've had to allow people to take my arm and guide me, which is very hard for me. People look at me and they know I have AIDS. Yet if I want to get from one place to another, I have to accept this help. As the disease progresses, you let people intrude more in your life. Formalizing some of these things, like arranging for a buddy, a home health aide, a house cleaner, a weekly nurse, making these things sort of official has helped and has taken the strain off friends.
>
> Another characteristic of the good patient is to have a realistic expectation of what your doctor will be able to do for you. My expectation has been that perhaps my doctors can manage this chronic disease which will involve a lot of hospitalizations, a lot of illnesses, and a lot of problems, while maintaining some quality of life. But I don't have any expectations that they can save my life. Certainly not any more. I often leave the doctor's office feeling they don't know a lot more than I do. My doctor has

said to me several times in the last year, "I don't know what to tell you" about a major decision. I guess a responsibility of the patient is to accept that or to change doctors—one or the other. You have to make peace with that, you know.*

The notion of survival as a function of faith in one's self is echoed by many patients. This is not to suggest the converse—that those who do not live a long time lacked faith in themselves nor does it mean that they necessarily lacked other characteristics of the effective patient. These attributes may promote well-being and longer survival but certainly are not in and of themselves sufficient to extend life.

BEHAVIORS AND ATTITUDES THAT MAY PROLONG LIFE

One patient offered these comments on the value of a positive attitude:

> Lots of things contribute to long-term survival, but one is a positive attitude. An attitude that there's more than you going through this, that there are people involved in your life whom you love, who love you, that there's a support system you really relate to and enjoy. And, that you have a working relationship with your doctors. You get to a place within yourself that you know what you want to do with your own health care, that there are certain things that feel better to you than other things. As long as you feel that way, it doesn't matter what the outcome is. You have love in your life and goals.

What Is a "Good Attitude" and Why Is It Important?

While difficult to define precisely, "good attitude" is the capacity to continue to anticipate future good times and to believe that your life is worth living, that your survival has meaning to yourself or others, that there are still things left for you to learn emotionally, intellectually, and spiritually. A positive attitude is the conviction that you have value, that you matter, that your life is worthwhile and is worth struggling to preserve.

People with positive attitudes certainly may feel enraged, devastated, heartbroken, and fearful at times; such feelings are inescapable, particularly in the face of chronic, serious illness and death. People with positive attitudes do get sick and die, but it is not because of their attitudes. Although long-term survival with HIV illness is not purely a function of a good attitude, the converse is usually the case: Those who are long-term survivors usually have faith in themselves and the value and meaning of their lives and have gone to great lengths to keep going.

---

*Comment: This man battled with progressive and finally total blindness, partial deafness, loss of balance, loss of bladder control, and increasing neuropathy that eventually confined him to bed, unable to turn over by himself. He died 6 months after this conversation, talking about new treatment options and alternative strategies to the very end. When he was finally put on I.V. morphine, he insisted on taking dextroamphetamine (Dexedrine) to keep himself alert when he was awake. He considered himself an indifferent patient, but his friends, and we, thought he was a champion.

Treatment for AIDS is often grueling, arduous, and unpleasant. Life has to be considered worthwhile to submit to 12 hours a day of I.V. feeding, for example. Eventually many things may have to be sacrificed in the struggle to stay alive with progressive illness. The driving force underlying that struggle is referred to as "attitude."

The Value of Social Ties

Like physicians, patients recognize the influence of social attachments on health and survival. Friends and family can provide good advice, humor, advocacy, and generally assist with concrete needs and services. Even the help of just one other person can be invaluable, particularly in a crisis.

For many, it's an issue of discovering who one's true friends are and investing in those important relationships. Others may find themselves having meaningful relationships that they've never experienced before: "I had no friendships before AIDS," one such person said. "I felt so totally different from everyone else. I worked, but I kept my employees and coworkers at arm's length. Because of AIDS, I've had more of a social life than before."

Unfortunately, the cost of having close relationships is the risk of losing them. As one long-term AIDS survivor said, "One of the hardest things is watching your friends die. That is the wearing part, the exhausting part. After a while it is grief beyond belief. And the longer you live with this thing, the more losses there are. There never seems to be a reward for being a long-term survivor…just prolonged grief."

Identity and Transformation

For many individuals living with HIV/AIDS, maintaining one's identity means continuing to do work that has always brought satisfaction and pride. For others, however, leaving a job and engaging in new activities brings greater satisfaction.

Confronting the challenges of HIV may bring about significant changes, including attitudes about living, lifestyle behaviors, inner strengths, prejudices, and communities that once felt foreign and strange. Living with HIV actually transforms some individuals, forcing them to define their goals and identities.

The discovery of HIV status sometimes has the impact of a religious conversion, transforming a life of addiction, prison, and disrupted relationships, to a stable, valued existence. A long-term survivor described the transformations in her life following her HIV diagnosis:

> I see life through different eyes today. I appreciate life now. Every day to me is like a new and exciting adventure. Every day that I have I'm grateful for, especially if I'm healthy.
>
> My perspective has changed a lot. I see challenges as an opportunity to do something. Before they were something I had to go through. I'm just grateful to be alive, grateful to be able to help somebody, grateful to have

another day. Things are different now than before.

My whole lifestyle has changed, too. I had to change my way of think-ing and change my attitude. That's been so hard. First I had to find help for the addiction. I was on drugs over 20 years, since I was 12. I knew I had to go somewhere and get help, and I did. I went to a 12-step program which I still go to today and will probably go to for the rest of my life.

Then I had to address the mental health issue. That was really impor-tant, too, I think. You know, why did I stick needles in my arms all them years? Something must have been going on.

And then there was a changing of my attitude—becoming more open. I was a member of ACT-UP. I had never been around gay men. Never in my life. But they were fighting for the same cause I was. They had been dealing with the same issues as me. And so it didn't matter that I was this girl from the Bronx coming down to Astor Place, at Cooper Union, and sit-ting there with all these people that were of a totally different experience, totally different world. We had something in common. Our hearts were in the same place.

First time I ever saw two men kissing, I thought, "What's happening here?" Then I realized that one of them was sick and the other one was his lover and was consoling him. And all I saw was love. So all those other notions I had started to dissipate, you know, and things just started changing. My heart became lighter.

There's been a change in my family setting. My children and I live together, and there's a real nice, warm home. There's a lot of dialogue, and a lot of love and support for each other. I'm able to help my son pay his col-lege tuition, where I couldn't do that before.

Keeping Busy and Setting Goals
Keeping busy is a way of surviving. But, more than remaining active for its own sake, there are tremendous psychological, and perhaps even physical, benefits to developing and maintaining specific goals when living with HIV. Goals may be relatively long-term, intermediate, or even very short-term. What's important is maintaining incentives to live, to feel that there's something left to accomplish or to learn or to contribute to the world.

WHY AREN'T ALL PATIENTS "GOOD" PATIENTS?
Inadequate medical care is one of the most significant barriers to being a good patient. Access to appropriate care is the first prerequisite. To some extent, this may not be within the patient's control, depending on finances, geog-raphy, and health insurance. Patients, however, need to recognize the importance of their role in identifying and obtaining the best health care that is possible. Often, because of cultural, socioeconomic, or personal factors, many patients do not see themselves as having any choice when it comes to where, how, and from whom they receive health care services. Since most patients are not as persistent as the woman described earlier in this chapter,

it's often helpful for a counselor or some other informed person to encourage and facilitate patient choice and action.

And, sometimes people can work together to obtain better care. For example, there is no major hospital in the area of Provincetown, Massachusetts. The Provincetown AIDS Support Group solved this problem by raising money to purchase a van. Community volunteers use the van at least once a week to drive people with HIV illness to the medical facilities in Boston.

"I Don't Want to Talk About It"
One man explained:

> The patient has to be able to articulate his problems because the doctor isn't going to be able to read his mind. That's a problem sometimes for me and my friends. The majority of people won't talk about their emotions or physical pain. They don't want to be sick, so they don't admit it to anyone, including their doctors. Some things like diarrhea and loss of bowel control are embarrassing to discuss. Talking about pain isn't so much embarrassing as it is difficult to acknowledge. It's hard to accept that you're not able to do certain things anymore. You become an expert at tuning it out. All of a sudden you can't tune it out any more, but the doctor isn't a mind reader.

Survivor "Guilt"
In the context of AIDS, survivor guilt generally refers to seronegative people whose friends, lovers, and community become sick around them. However, it also has meaning for people who have HIV infection but who live longer or stay healthier than others who became infected at the same time or subsequently.

One patient, who lived for 6 years after he was first diagnosed with PCP, was the only one left in his support group. Not only did the original members die but also all the people who had joined in subsequent years. He actually said, "I feel survivor guilt myself in the face of all these friends who have died recently. I would go see them with rosy cheeks and a bounce in my step and I couldn't help but feel them glaring at me, 'What's he doing that I'm not?'"

Another PWA stopped taking care of himself because his lover, who seroconverted after he did, was declining more rapidly. So he stopped working out, stopped trying to eat carefully, stopped the meditation he had found soothing. Only after his lover had died and he noticed he was still feeling reasonably good, did it occur to him that he had been trying to minimize the difference in health status between them by neglecting himself.

Not Trusting Physicians
Patients, like physicians, generally recognize that honesty is essential in the doctor-patient relationship and is seen as a reflection of trust in the physi-

cian. One patient who worked at a social service agency for HIV clients observed, "There's a certain type of person who is terrified. These patients panic and don't believe that anyone can help them. They try a couple of doctors, but they don't tell one about the other. All of their common sense goes out the window and fear takes over. They just don't believe any doctor is going to help, and they don't trust anybody. The one person you've got to trust in all this is your doctor. If you don't trust him, then you don't have anything."

Little Faith in Treatment

There may come a time when the patient concludes that there are no remaining medical solutions. One man expressed his feelings at this stage poignantly: "We AIDS patients go into these physicians' offices with an expectation that they're going to cure or solve our illnesses. We were raised that way. Is that completely ridiculous of us? We have the expectation that doctors will make us better, but in fact they can't. It's not because they don't want to. They just can't. They may even look at us and think we are ludicrous to come in with this expectation."

A time may come when some patients wonder if they want to spend their remaining time "sitting in an empty room looking at a bottle dripping." They may prefer to discontinue treatments and engage in more pleasurable activities. One patient said, "I certainly know people with AIDS who spent their last year doing what they enjoyed, instead [of continuing with treatment]. That's a valid idea to me. I probably won't know until the time comes if I'm glad or sorry I've stuck to treatments."

When illness persists unremittingly, and the physician cannot offer additional remedies, some people will shed the role of patient and discontinue their medical care (except for comfort). As will be discussed in some detail in Chapter 11, we do not regard this decision as a personal failure of any kind. We believe it is the right of each individual to decide when to redirect attention from conquering illness to living and dying with as much grace and comfort as possible. At that point, the patient role may no longer be relevant.

4

WHAT MAKES A GOOD HIV SPECIALIST?

COMMENT

While physicians and patients would agree on many of the qualities of the ideal HIV specialist, contrasting needs and roles will occasionally result in different priorities. Certain characteristics, such as competence and medical expertise, for example, are universally desired; other traits, such as type of office practice or sexual orientation, are more likely to be a matter of "fit" between patient and physician. While office location, for example, may seem rather insignificant to a physician, proximity to home may become paramount to a decreasingly mobile and increasingly home-bound patient. And, regardless of a physician's credentials and experience, if patients cannot reach the doctor, they may feel abandoned and uncared for. Thus, the question of what makes a "good" HIV specialist must be approached from both the professional's and patient's perspectives.

COMPETENCE AND COMPASSION

An ethicist who studied physicians and patients observed that

> Two excellences or "virtues" are popularly held as appropriate to and necessary for physicians: competence and compassion. Competence for physicians takes two forms. One component would include those capacities grounded in medical knowledge and its application: diagnosis and treatment. A second component could be characterized as nonmedical though traditionally associated in an inseparable way with the physician's role: understanding, sympathy, comfort, patience. A second premier excellence for physicians is compassion, understood as a sympathy for the distress of another with a desire to help. Compassion is not a relic that remains from the period of medicine's impotence. It is a central pillar upon which patient-physician relationships are built (Shelp, 1984, p 352).

AIDS is unlike other illnesses because of the severity, number, and variety of progressive, often life-threatening diseases treated with multiple toxic medications that require close and ongoing monitoring. Consequently, HIV patients see far more of their physicians over a longer period of time than the average patient, and for more serious problems. Although all patients seek competent physicians, regardless of how infrequently they are consulted, compassion is most relevant in cases of chronic illness.

The needs of AIDS patients are thus qualitatively, as well as medically, unusual. Compassion and related qualities like trust, communication, and accessibility become essential. Outstanding HIV specialists also are creative and aggressive in their approach to treatment, helping the patient plan for change throughout the disease course and facilitating home treatment when possible.

CURING VERSUS HEALING

In understanding what makes a good HIV specialist, it is also helpful to consider the distinction between "illness," which refers to objective disease that physicians seek to "cure" by technical medical methods, and "sickness," which is a subjective state that can be "healed" (Cassell, 1976).

$$\left.\begin{array}{l} \text{ILLNESS} \\[1em] \text{DISEASE} \end{array}\right\} \rightarrow \text{CURE}$$

$$\text{SICKNESS} \rightarrow \text{HEALING}$$

A person can be ill (e.g., with diabetes, hypertension, or cancer) and not even be aware of the disease. However, one cannot be sick without knowing it. Sickness entails feeling disconnected from the world (the healthy world), losing one's usual sense of indestructibility, and having a perception of diminished personal control. These manifestations or "symptoms" of sickness can be healed, at least to some extent, even if the illness cannot be cured or, indeed, progresses.

Although healing can be effectively performed by nonphysicians and indeed by nonmedical people, it has always been an integral part of medicine. For most of history, medical cures were absent. However, since the 1930s when the sulfonamides were discovered to treat bacterial infections, enormous progress has been made in the discovery and development of cures for many diseases. But there has been a corresponding decline in the attention and energy devoted to the practice of healing.

Western medicine and an informed, experienced physician are needed to cure complicated diseases like those associated with HIV infection. In addition, a caring, compassionate practitioner is needed to heal the patient, even when cure is not possible. It is important to recognize the difference. Because both disease and sickness are components of HIV illness, the ability to heal as well as cure is an essential attribute of an effective HIV physician.

PHYSICIAN PERSPECTIVES

THE "GOOD" HIV SPECIALIST

- Experience with HIV
- Interpersonal skills
- Hospital affiliation
- Primary care orientation
- Ability to arrange and manage home care
- Vigilance
- Willingness to help patients understand and negotiate the health care system
- Sensitivity to the uncertainties and anxieties of HIV illness

---

Experience with HIV

Knowledge and experience go together. There are few authoritative textbooks on the treatment of AIDS-related problems because new findings make textbooks rapidly obsolete and because there are no standard treatments for a considerable number of AIDS-related conditions. Consequently, experience is the basic source of knowledge, including familiarity with signs and symptoms of HIV illness, and currently available procedures, interventions, standards of treatment, and the current research literature.

People living with HIV/AIDS cannot afford to seek care from a physician who may be otherwise competent but is not familiar with the general terrain of HIV disease. The chances are too great that important problems will be missed. When there is an option—and there almost always is—it is best to look for a primary care provider who has accumulated significant experience in providing direct HIV care, has trained in an HIV care setting, or is affiliated with colleagues who have considerable experience treating people with HIV. If a health care provider says that he or she doesn't need to know that much about HIV and its associated illnesses to provide good health care to an HIV-infected person, another provider should be sought.

Interpersonal Skills

Physicians, like patients, emphasize interpersonal skills as an essential aspect of being good at AIDS medicine. The effective or "good" doctor is one who takes the trouble to talk to people, who is sensitive to personal issues raised by patients, who has the time to sit down and listen to patients, and who will treat patients as individuals, not merely "charts" or cases. As one physician noted, "Knowledge is useless without humanity."

The role of kindness was stressed by many physicians:

> It's amazing to me how many people continue to go to doctors who treat them unkindly. I think it's appalling. For example, I know an infectious dis-

ease specialist who is unbelievably smart, and I call him for all kinds of questions. I think he's brilliant, but I wouldn't send him a friend with HIV disease because I don't think he's that nice to people. I'd send a friend for a diagnostic dilemma but not for ongoing care.

Another physician elaborated on what he meant by compassion:

When I refer a patient I want someone accessible, sensitive, and spiritual. The role of the AIDS doctor goes beyond medicine. He is going to be taking care of the patient, most likely, in the last moments. Now is that going to be done with the doctor's head in the chart, or will he hold the patient's hand and take care of mom as well?

Also important is commitment to working with AIDS and the people who have AIDS. One physician felt strongly that, "Someone with HIV disease should go to doctors who have committed themselves to an ongoing relationship with this disease. The doctor's sexual orientation doesn't matter but I think patients should run as fast as they can from any doctor who even hints at disapproval of alternate lifestyles."

Hospital Affiliation

In general, physicians feel that hospital affiliation is important. Although some experienced and respected HIV physicians do not have any hospital affiliation, for the most part hospital privileges are necessary. As one physician said, "It is inevitable in the history of any given HIV patient's disease that hospitalization will be required."

A Primary Care Orientation

The ability to see the big picture and to treat the patient as a whole enhances medical management. One physician expressed this in terms of "having a primary care orientation, which means focusing on the needs of the patient rather than on the specific illness."

Home Care

One of the major gains in AIDS care during the last decade is better management of opportunistic infections and secondary illnesses, which can now often be treated on an outpatient basis. Although hospitalization is sometimes unavoidable, home care is often feasible and preferred. The chronicity of HIV illness, the range of conditions that may occur over time, and increasing third-party restrictions on duration of hospital stays create the opportunity and the need for treatment in the home setting. New technologies in home care have also altered the practice of AIDS primary care.

With some exceptions, most acutely ill HIV patients prefer to be treated at home rather than in the hospital. And even from a medical standpoint, it may be safer for a patient with a suppressed immune system to avoid hospitals because of nosocomial (hospital-induced) infections and contagious diseases like tuberculosis. Some patients wish to avoid the hospital because of past experience with unsympathetic staff who do not want to work with AIDS patients. For others, home care is preferable because of the opportunity to remain in a familiar, comfortable environment with considerably more personal control.

Home care can, however, present a tremendous logistic as well as clinical challenge to the HIV physician. For the HIV specialist who is already overscheduled, arranging the myriad details of home care can be overwhelming. It is much easier if all patients are in the same hospital, where the physician is not responsible for nursing coverage, delivery of medical supplies, and coordination of health and support services. In the hospital, the physician can stop by daily or more often and see how the patient looks and what is happening. And, these visits are reimbursed in full by insurance. In contrast, management of a patient at home, where skilled nursing care is needed, usually means multiple telephone calls at all hours of the day and night should plans go awry (and they often do), as well as paperwork, for which the physician is not reimbursed. Since daily visits are not practical, it is necessary to rely on the home care nurses for reports of the patient's condition. Plans of care must be discussed with the field staff, who may have little expertise in treating HIV illness. This is often complicated by high staff turnover, requiring the physician to repeat information that he or she has already communicated. The physician also must coordinate laboratory tests and services provided by multiple agencies, all with similar but not identical requirements and policies. Altogether, home care is time-consuming, complicated, and more subject to problems than is hospital care.

The Physician's Contributions to Long-Term Survival
The physician contributes to survival by providing quality HIV medical care, which includes "being meticulous and up to date" and "being on top of things and getting people in promptly, when they're ill." An important part of this expert care consists of the timely initiation of appropriate prophylactic treatment.

Vigilance. Diagnosing illnesses and opportunistic infections early and treating them appropriately and aggressively is a hallmark of excellent HIV care and occurs most readily when both patient and physician are vigilant. One physician said, "In caring for AIDS patients, you have to be very quick on the draw. If a patient calls and says that he has a headache and fever, he has to be seen right away. We've learned to recognize relevant symptoms and evaluate patients very quickly." Another physician explained, "There are doctors who do better than others, because of experience and attitude. A patient who comes in with clear-cut PCP [*Pneumocystis carinii* pneumonia] symptoms could wind up being treated for bronchitis by an inexperienced clinician. Physicians may delay diagnosis or unintentionally mask a diagnosis by giving an antibiotic for every fever, which makes finding MAI [*Myobacterium avium intracellulare*] difficult."

Education. Physicians can also contribute to survival by educating patients about medical procedures. Part of this entails encouraging a sense of participation and partnership. In addition, preparing patients for specific medical procedures reduces anxiety. One physician felt it was important to explain and describe the system for patients "so that when they go for an MRI [imaging procedure], they know that they're going to be in a weird tube. Or, if I'm ordering a zillion tests, I let them know about this. Or, if they're going to meet a doctor who has an edgy personality, but is very good technically, I will tell them, this is what he's like as a person...."

Another physician spoke of how important it is to not assume understanding on the part of the patient:

> An oncologist once described having cancer as parachuting into a jungle without a map or a compass. That must be what it's like to have an uncharted disease. Often I assume that patients understand, when actually they don't. When I worked with patients who were political activists or who were physicians themselves, I used to think, "I won't explain that, they know that." I realize now that's absolutely untrue. So, now I tell patients how I've reached a decision, and they really appreciate that. It doesn't matter how smart they are.

This style of interaction on the part of the physician provides reassurance and comfort as much as concrete information. It seems likely, also, that it enhances patient compliance with difficult and often anxiety-provoking procedures that may be a necessary part of quality care.

Dealing with the Uncertainty of HIV Disease

One of the more challenging tasks for physicians, as well as other professionals who work with HIV patients, is to help people anticipate what lies ahead. No one can predict how an individual case will evolve. People who are still well often ask how much time they have before the onset of symptoms or infections. Some people, especially when first tested, ask whether illness is inevitable. Is it appropriate for the professional to say, "Who knows? You may never get sick. Nobody can tell when scientists will make a breakthrough"? If this answer is given, it is usually with the intention of offering hope and an incentive to cope. In this, as in many other aspects of HIV care, there are no absolute answers.

Most physicians stress the value of communicating optimism during the early stages of the infection. In general, people are encouraged to go about their daily lives. Of course, some issues should be addressed, such as choosing a physician and assessing insurance needs, which itself might entail decisions about job changes, disability, and so on. Some physicians feel this is an appropriate time—before the person gets sick—to address the "paperwork" of death (health proxies, wills, "do not resuscitate" orders, funeral arrangements). "I always tell people right away when they are HIV-positive, 'Listen. We should all have a living will, we should all know exactly what we want. The biggest problem is losing control. So you take care of it all now, you put it in a box, you put it away, and you go back to work. You know everything is in that box.'" Other physicians, however, prefer to wait until later in the disease course to bring up this subject.

Even when an AIDS-defining condition is diagnosed, most physicians feel that an encouraging tone is appropriate. For example, one physician explained, "If they are newly diagnosed with PCP, I tell them I'm fairly confident that we can maintain a good quality of life for 2 or 3 years, and with prayers and hope and good luck perhaps by then we will have a better handle on things. I think this is honest. It's what I like to think."

Another physician offered the following approach:

> Many people have asked me, "How much time do I have?" Let's say somebody has 20 T4 cells. I will say, "Well, things have changed. It used to be that the majority of people lived less than a year. Most people now live 2 years, and I know occasional people who live 3 or 4 years. But they are the exceptions." And that's usually a good enough answer for people. They will not ask you much more than that.

Physicians are often reluctant to cite illness statistics as a way of helping patients understand what to expect. In fact, one suggested doing the opposite:

> I don't think it helps at all to say, "With a diagnosis of X, there is a 62% chance you'll be dead in 6 months." It just doesn't pay. I always say to people, "You know all about the statistics," even if they don't. "So let me tell you about the 20% of people from the San Francisco Men's Health Project who are asymptomatic after 10 years." Everyone knows the bad stuff, but not everyone knows the other side of it.

PATIENT PERSPECTIVES

> What I like best about my doctor is that she's well informed. She doesn't just sit down and prescribe things for me. We have conversations. She gives me different options. Ultimately, I make the choice about what I'm going to take. I don't feel like she thinks she knows it all. I feel like we work together. I also feel that she's very sensitive and humorous. She's very respectful. She treats people with dignity. She takes time with people to explain things. Those are the qualities that I see in her and that I like about her.

The characteristics of the "good" HIV physician as described by experienced patients are not very different from those given by physicians. They include practical considerations, such as being knowledgeable and having expertise about HIV disease; behavioral factors, such as taking the time to explain things; willingness to participate in a "partnership" with the patient; and being sensitive and caring. Many AIDS long-term survivors ultimately find one physician with whom they are tremendously satisfied—a physician they respect and feel respected by, whose expertise they trust and admire, and who is supportive, encouraging, and cares about them. They often attribute their survival, at least in part, to their relationship with their physician.

The criteria and qualities most often mentioned by patients in defining what makes a good HIV specialist were:

- Hospital affiliation
- How the office practice is organized and managed
- Creativity and assertiveness
- Communication
- Encouragement, compassion, and understanding

The Medical Practice

Even if a physician is a superb clinician, the medical needs of HIV extend beyond the individual. And while affiliation and practice structure would appear to be within the province of physicians, how a medical practice is set up can significantly affect the quality of a patient's experience.

Hospital Affiliation and Referrals. Patients give various reasons for hospital preferences, including geographic location (i.e., near home, in a preferred neighborhood), physical accommodations, and, probably most important, the hospital's reputation for HIV/AIDS care.

If a physician does not have admitting privileges at any hospital, the patient may be referred to a municipal hospital, with its own staff, or another physician may have to admit the patient and be responsible for him or her on a daily basis. When the original primary care provider is not involved, the result can be fragmented care.

Referrals to Specialists. Almost as important as the physician's own level of HIV experience is his or her ability to coordinate referrals to experienced and knowledgeable subspecialists. As illnesses develop, such subspecialty skills as oncology or gastroenterology are often required for optimal care.

Office Management. Although hospital affiliation is a central issue during periods of acute illness, people are seen most often in the office as outpatients. A well-run and well-staffed office can make a huge difference in the experience of being a patient. Simple courtesies by staff as well as physician, such as being greeted by name and hearing some expression of personal interest, are particularly appreciated when visits are frequent. Patients also mention the importance of getting timely and effective help with paperwork for insurance reimbursement and benefits, which may require frequent resubmissions.

In many busy offices, a particular staff member may play a central role in relating to patients, helping to solve problems, and facilitating access to the physician. Sometimes, simple friendliness and humor help reduce tension. One man said, "When I go see Dr. X, I am so anxious and upset. And there's this long wait, and I get more anxious the longer I wait. But when Julio is there at the desk, we talk about his love affairs and all of his adventures, and it's always like a soap opera. I laugh and relax and feel okay by the time I see the doctor."

Telephone Calls. Getting through to the physician by telephone, or being able to leave an urgent message, is critical, according to patients. No one who is sick or frightened wants to hear a taped recording, "The office is closed until tomorrow and this machine takes no messages." Another issue that is particularly important to patients is the length of time it takes for the physician to return calls. Those who have experienced (or have been present when someone they care about has experienced) new and frightening symptoms that cause severe distress or seem to signal an impending medical disaster can appreciate the tension of waiting by the telephone for the physician to return a call. This may take hours or, in some cases, even days, even when the physician is not out of town. On the other hand, HIV specialists may get literally dozens of calls in a day (not only from patients but from nurses in home care situations, pharmacies, insurance representatives, and quality assurance personnel in hospitals). No matter how much time may be allocated for returning calls, it is never quite enough. In the most efficient medical practices, an experienced assistant screens calls, transmits messages, and even returns calls about simple matters. The routine is distinguished from the urgent, and the physician is freer to concentrate on situations that require his or her intervention.

Coverage and Availability. Physicians differ widely in their personal availability, both during and after office hours. Some have younger associates who are likely to see new patients. Others feel that referrals come to them because of their personal reputation and that seeing such patients should not be delegated. After hours, some share coverage and others do not.

Creativity and Assertiveness
Since the problems of HIV infection are new to Western medicine, management of the disease requires creativity and an assertive approach. In the absence of cures, persistence and innovation are welcomed by patients:

> What I like most about my physician is that he's creative. He's never said, "It can't be done, there's nothing I can do for you." He always seems to have a solution. It may not be orthodox, but it's something. He knows a lot about research. He seems to know what's happening in the AIDS community. And he taps a lot of resources. He doesn't say, "Well, you've got this and there's nothing I can do about it." He'll go as far as he can to get a clear diagnosis and then he'll try something. It may not work but still he gave it a shot. You feel if something doesn't work, at least he left no stone unturned.

Communication
To establish a good relationship, the physician needs to take the time to provide explanations to the patient. While assertiveness by the patient plays a role, the physician must believe in the merit of informing patients and

involving them in their own care. He or she must be willing to invest time and effort explaining office procedures and coverage, philosophy of care, rationale for different treatment strategies, diagnostic and treatment procedures, and what to expect from treatment. Unfortunately, some of the best HIV physicians are so busy that time for patients always seems limited. "My major complaint," said one patient of his physician, "is that his practice is too big, and although I consider him to be a good doctor, I need more time with him; it's been a constant source of frustration."

Ironically, it's easier for patients to insist on adequate explanations from their physicians when they're feeling well. When they're experiencing pain, fatigue, or an acute illness, patients must rely on the physician to initiate explanations. "What's good about my doctor is that she takes the time to explain things—if I pin her down. But that's the problem: As I get weaker, I find myself less able to pin her down." At such times, the otherwise "vigilant" patient may not have the energy or ability to ask all of the important questions.

A Good Listener. The flip side of providing information is being a good listener. Although all patients like to feel they are being listened to, this may be a particularly important skill with an illness such as HIV, which is fraught with uncertainty. Patients have worries and apprehensions that need airing. Trust in the doctor-patient relationship is particularly important in later-stage disease, when patients often feel less in control and more in need of someone who knows and respects their wishes and desires. Sometimes, at the end, being a listener, a "witness," is the most valuable service that one can offer.

Encouragement, Compassion, and Understanding

If faith in one's treatment plays a role in the effectiveness of that treatment, as many believe, the physician can, by his or her encouragement, affect the outcome of treatment. Moreover, a pat on the back by one's physician can be extraordinarily meaningful. "He always tells me that I'm a great patient and he's very proud of me," an appreciative patient remarked.

Another patient described how his physician kept him from giving up when he felt defeated:

> Recently, there have been times, I will admit, when I want to pack it all in. I get so tired of being a receptacle for drugs. I just want to take all those bottles of pills and throw them in the trash, lay back, and let nature take its course. And my doctor always sighs and says, "I wouldn't advise that, Raymond. It's a possible course of action, but I wouldn't advise it. You and I both know what course nature would take and fairly quickly."

In addition to support and encouragement, patients appreciate physicians who are concerned about them as individuals. One man explained,

> The first thing that comes to mind, which may sound silly, is that he always puts his arm around me at the end of the visit, which may not sound like

anything but I feel that he really likes me and really cares about me, and that he doesn't mix my file up with someone who has a similar name, or he doesn't only vaguely know who I am. You may wait 3 hours to see him, but when you see him he is 100% there with you. Office visits are very long and very thorough.

THE DOCTOR-PATIENT MATCH

Physicians often point out that a good patient is only half of the equation that comprises the doctor-patient relationship. "There's a difference between what is a good patient in the abstract and what is *my* good patient," one doctor said. "I think there are different types of people and when they find their own best style of doctor, there's a melding of personalities. Since I'm pretty aggressive, I attract a certain type of patient whereas I'm going to scare away another type. You want to work with someone that you can get along with, that you enjoy, and vice versa." In view of the long-term nature of relationships with HIV and people, the match between physician and patient is critical for both to be maximally effective.

Some patients may be particularly drawn to physicians who are comfortable combining conventional and alternative treatment strategies. While almost no one refuses to let their patients engage in alternative therapies as long as they do not preclude standard treatments, some are more enthusiastic about them than others.

Staying the Course

Patients are often concerned about being abandoned, particularly if they become terminally ill. "Ultimately, it's not the fact that I will die of this that bothers me nor am I afraid of death itself. It's the process of dying of AIDS and of being abandoned that really frightens me. I want to know that my doctor will not abandon me if he feels like there's nothing left to do or because I don't have any money or insurance left." Such reassurance can help patients cope with fears of an agonizing and undignified death.

WHAT PATIENTS WANT TO HEAR...
WHAT PHYSICIANS ARE WILLING TO SAY

Patients want their physicians to be open, communicative, and frank about their beliefs regarding diagnosis, treatment, and, most importantly, what they do and do not know about HIV illness. Patients also want their physicians to be hopeful...yet realistic. Striking an appropriate balance may be quite difficult. As one patient said, "He's not pessimistic. He's very even tempered, although he's not overly optimistic either. He's never given me any false promises or miracles. He's skeptical, but on some level optimistic."

Both patients and physicians praise the virtue of honesty, but they sometimes disagree about just *how* honest the physician should be. Physicians generally say they emphasize the positive and are, if anything, unduly optimistic up to the point where significant deterioration occurs. However, patients are apt to perceive the converse. In describing a conversation with his physician, one long-term survivor provided an example of the delicate balance the physician faces in trying to be candid and at the same time encouraging. He had just described at length how wonderful he thought his physician was, how caring and helpful. When asked about any problems, he gave this answer:

> Sometimes I want to ask him, "Am I going to make it? Am I going to pull through this illness and be better?" And I don't ask him that question because I feel it's unfair, that it puts him in an untenable position. So I've tried not to ask him, but occasionally I wouldn't mind a little more encouragement. This is true in my life in general…sometimes you wish people would encourage you even if they're lying. For example, for people to say, "You're going to be fine. Don't worry, they'll find a cure, you'll be all right, just hang in there a few more years." Nobody ever really said that because there's such a widespread reluctance to be naive or "pollyannish." Nobody wants to sound false in that way.
>
> I asked the doctor if I should go to graduate school or make long-term plans like that, and that was sort of a sneaky way of asking him, "Do I have a future?" And he said, "Yes. You should definitely go to graduate school." But then he said, "If something changes, then we'll adjust to that." So I got a sort of 50/50 answer and I would have liked something more, even if he didn't really believe it. That caveat attached to his answer really made me feel discouraged about making long-term plans.

Another very articulate PWA listened to this passage and commented as follows:

> What's nice about my doctor is that I think I'm up on everything, and he will come up with something that hasn't been published yet, and I haven't heard of yet. I'll hear about it maybe a month after he's told me and he was accurate. But I get the 50-50s, too, from him, and I don't really push it anymore because I don't want the 50-50s. I deal with the immediate with him.

[Interviewer: Well, what's a doctor to do?]

> Oh, sometimes I think it would be very good to just go into a flight of fantasy with the patients and—like graduate school—say, "Yeah, sure, GO to graduate school." You might not take anything on because you [worry that you] could be hit by a car. Anyone could be hit by a car. So, I mean, you have to rearrange everything, but unless you are hit by a car, you're going to finish graduate school. I sometimes think doctors are too scrupulous and are not leaving enough up to God, to fate, to whatever. Maybe you will get through graduate school and maybe it's just the long-term goal you need to carry you through. I really do believe that long-term goals are important.

Physicians who read both these patient interviews commented as follows:

The first physician answered rather briefly,

> I am not fanciful. People ask me, "Are they going to have a cure for this disease?" And I simply say "No." I have a real hard opinion on that and I just tell people, there is no cure for this disease. It's going to go the way of smallpox. It's going to have to be extinguished over time. And the population affected is going to die of the disease. And that's how it is.

The second physician stated,

> I would say that those two patients could very well have come from my practice.... Basically I try to encourage people—it sounds so trite—to live for the day. But not to be unrealistic about changes. And then you adapt and adjust. It seems to me that these two people want to hear a flight of fancy. But I'd bet that those two people wouldn't be happy if they really thought their doctor was being too flip in terms of the positive. Part of what I read in there is that they're comfortable with the fact that their doctors are not going to limit their possibilities except with what could be realistic limitations. I think that's all you have to do. That's just life.

The third physician said,

> The patient puts a lot of trust in me as the physician and trusts that I am going to be honest with him. And so if I were very misleading, way down the line it could backfire. I tell patients, "You can almost turn this around to your advantage. So many people go through life not appreciating each day, and it's important to live more for the day. And I also tell them they should do with their life what they want to do, and I encourage them not so much to make long-range plans as to go on with life. Sometimes patients will set up a goal with the idea that nothing can happen until that goal is achieved. But I try to discourage them if it seems overwhelming.... I have patients who ask me "Am I going to make it?" I remind them of multiple different options. I'll say something like, "AZT has been shown to give you 7 months of life; if you do prophylaxis, that'll give you more time; who knows what's going to be available then—that's the kind of picture I paint. I just think my role is to be honest, not cruel, but honest with the patient—that's what trust is.

The last physician offered a more complex response:

> I encourage people to make long-term plans and to travel and to take new jobs. When life deals you a terrible blow, that can be a time when you reevaluate and decide what's important.... And I do say to people, "All you have to do is stay well, stay stable for a few more years until there is a combination of drugs that puts you into remission. I don't know if there'll be a cure in your lifetime, but I'm hoping that you can remain well long enough—with a combination of good treatments and taking really good care of yourself—to take advantage of any drugs that might be developed."

Do I believe it? Some days I do and some days I don't. Today I don't but last week when I had a good day or two, I believed it. If you had said to me 10 years ago, "In your lifetime you'll see people with HIV survive for years and years," I would have said, "You're nuts." So we've made a lot of progress, although obviously not enough. That's my most optimistic view of things. But, my patients are really smart. And I'm not going to feed them B.S., because then I'm not credible.

These physicians are not willing to join their patients in denial. And while they encourage optimism and long-range planning, they seem to feel that their role is to help patients remain realistic. Patients, on the other hand, may at times engage in a sort of magical thinking. "If the doctor would only say, 'Don't worry. You'll be all right,' then I will be." Unfortunately and ironically, if physicians gave patients what they say they want, the very foundation of the relationship—honesty—might be undermined and even irreparably damaged.

REFERENCES

Shelp EE. Courage: A neglected virtue in the patient-physician relationship. *Social Science and Medicine*. 1984;18:351-360.

Cassell E. *The Healer's Art*. Philadelphia: Lippincott; 1976.

5

THE DOCTOR-PATIENT RELATIONSHIP

COMMENT

The concept of egalitarian relationships between physicians and patients is fairly recent and is practiced perhaps nowhere as earnestly as in HIV medicine. Politically active, informed, and articulate gay men with AIDS—although suffering from a chronic and progressively debilitating disease—were not willing to participate in traditional paternalistic doctor-patient relationships. Thanks to their proactive stance, other patients with chronic, life-threatening diseases are learning to demand a full partnership with physicians in their own care.

TRADITIONAL DOCTOR-PATIENT ROLES

Traditionally, the roles of physicians and patients are perceived as fixed, static, and unequal. The physician is the wise, informed, knowledgeable, paternal expert who will cure rather than heal, whereas the patient is passive and obedient. In the traditional model of reciprocal obligations and privileges, the patient's obligations are (1) to be motivated to get well, (2) to seek technically competent help, and (3) to trust the physician. The physician's obligations are (1) to act for the patient's welfare, (2) to be guided by rules of professional behavior, (3) to be skilled and knowledgeable, and (4) to be objective and emotionally detached (Parsons, 1951).

These roles distribute authority unequally. The physician's position and leverage are "generated by professional prestige and situational authority of the health agent and situational dependency of the patient." The relative inequality of these positions is reinforced by the adoption of the sick role in which the patient "feels himself at least temporarily less than whole, weakened, open to fear and trembling" (Bloom and Wilson, 1979, p 275).

OTHER MODELS OF DOCTOR-PATIENT INTERACTION

In the 1950s, when psychiatrists became interested in the doctor-patient relationship, three different models were proposed (Szasz and Hollender, 1956): activity-passivity, guidance-cooperation, and mutual participation. In the activity-passivity model, the physician is in absolute control, and the patient is passive. Such a model is appropriate for emergencies and severe illnesses in which the patient is unable to participate in planning or choices, and the doctor is totally in charge. When HIV patients are very ill in either a resolving or terminal episode, and no loved one is present, this is the role the physician must assume.

The guidance-cooperation model is basically the "traditional" model of reciprocal obligations and privileges described above. It is appropriate in moderately severe acute and infectious disorders (Szasz and Hollender, 1956). The patient is ill, but alert, and is capable of exercising some judgment. Nevertheless, in this model, the patient is expected to accept the physician's authority and to carry out his or her instructions. With respect to the course of HIV illness, this is when patients start getting sick, often with an opportunistic infection. They may recover fully and return to work, or gradually restrict their lives according to their physical capacities. This "middle" stage may last for years.

In the model of mutual participation, doctors and patients are approximately equal in power; physicians help patients to help themselves. This approach is most often seen when a patient has a chronic illness "in which the treatment program is carried out by the patient with only occasional consultation with a physician. It requires a complex psychological and social organization on the part of the patient" (Bloom, 1963, p 41). This model is currently advocated by many academicians and AIDS activists who emphasize that equality is an essential component of an effective doctor-patient relationship.

The mutual participation model has become widely accepted by experts and is thus altering the nature of doctor-patient transactions. This is true of American medicine in general and of HIV medicine in particular. It has become the model of choice, in the absence of compelling reasons for either of the other two models (although these continue to have their place). In fact, patients are now expected to take more responsibility in managing their illnesses, and medical schools are training students to include patients in medical care decisions to an extent unheard of previously.

Of course, the doctor-patient relationship does not exist in a vacuum. Changing social realities, such as health care reform, as well as evolving technology, influence the nature of the interaction between patients and providers. The emergence of managed care and preferred providers has imposed limitations on the patient's freedom of choice of physicians and medical facilities and the doctor's choice about treatment type and duration. New expectations about informed consent, malpractice litigation, and evolving medical technologies, on the other hand, have led to a transformation of the doctor-patient relationship. Doctors are now motivated to obtain more careful informed consent from patients, which means disclosure of risks as well as benefits, and alternatives to the proposed treatment. One result is more dialogue and interaction than was formerly thought necessary. In addition, some responsibility has been transferred to the patient.

The availability of new technologies, in contrast, reduces the physician's need to talk to the patient; he or she can look at films and laboratory reports to diagnose and monitor disorders. As a professor of history and social medicine stated, "Technology placed doctors' hands more often on dials than on patients. Pausing by the bedside has become closer to being, diagnostically speaking, an indulgence, for the patient is frequently less interesting and less revealing about his symptoms than the technology" (Rothman, 1991).

CARVING OUT A PARTNERSHIP

A more direct source of the change in doctor-patient transactions in HIV medicine derives from the philosophies, attitudes, and assumptions about authority and responsibility of activists within the gay community. In the face of slow government response and inadequate provision of medical and social services, gay men initiated research, provided social services, and by becoming politically active, promoted necessary medical services for people with HIV illness. The early activists were smart and well-educated and often held high-level positions in business and various professions. They were fighting for their lives and the survival of their community. In this context, gay men with AIDS were not willing to assume the traditional docile, passive patient role; they demanded, and generally were granted, more participation in their medical care. This proactive stance is now being adopted by other people living with AIDS, as well as by patients with such diseases as breast cancer.

When both the patient and physician are engaged in care, the odds are greater that important signs and symptoms will not be missed. One specialist explained, "I think if you have a good relationship with your patients they are more likely to keep you informed of any developing problems and to be seen in a timely fashion."

Many HIV doctors insist that their patients become active partners in their own care.

> I think that patients who are active in their care are much more likely to do well than patients who come from the old school: "Just heal me; I'm just sort of a passing bystander and you give me pills." I sometimes have to take a patient and wake him up by saying, "I'm not going to do this to you, you're going to do it with me." I enjoy educating them, but it has some funny repercussions. I had a patient who grew up in a family where you went to the doctor and he gave you a shot and some pills and you never had to participate. He was very reluctant to get involved in his care. He never knew what medicines he was taking and what they were for. When he was in the hospital, I said, "I'm not going to let you leave until you can tell me what medications you're on, their names, the doses, and what they're for, and you're going to have to memorize them." Here's a guy who could speak four languages, but he refused to confront taking these medicines; but he learned, and now he's a very good patient.

Advantages of Equal Partnership

One of the consequences of mutual participation and teamwork between doctors and patients is a more realistic appraisal by the patient of what the physician can do.

A physician who was infected in 1983 wrote movingly of his relationship with his HIV specialist after 8 years:

> Sometimes, even my kind and dedicated doctor nearly lost hope. Two years ago, for example, I was hospitalized three times within a 2-month period. My blood counts were too low to tolerate the additional drop in leukocytes that the needed medications would cause. We were running out of options for my treatment. I could see in my old friend's eyes that he was feeling defeated. It was my turn to instill in him the "no reason to quit now" attitude. At that moment, it became clearer to me that the relationship between doctor and patient must be a reciprocal one. The doctor gives his or her best in taking care of the patient; the patient, whenever his or her condition allows, must provide feedback and participation in his or her own care, not as a passive recipient of services but rather as a protagonist in the struggle to achieve a better state of health (Aoun, 1992).

Learning from the Patient

Although in theory, most doctors endorse mutual participation, in practice there may be problems, at least the first time a physician encounters a patient who expects such a scenario. Physician identity, according to Parsons (1951), is partially based on special skills and knowledge. It is one thing to democratically share knowledge with the patient. It is quite another to face a patient who knows more than you do, at least about his or her disease. However, many AIDS specialists have come to appreciate and welcome the opportunity to learn from their patients. One relatively young physician described her experiences this way:

> One of the amazing things about working with HIV patients was the discovery that patients had read things I hadn't read and that they knew about scientific theories I didn't know about. In the beginning, I was worried they wouldn't respect me, and my feathers were ruffled a little bit.
>
> I worked with one man who was a brilliant immunologist. He would come in with stacks of articles from esoteric immunology journals and show them to me. I understood in the abstract. But then he would say, "What do you think?" and I'd say, "This is a little over my head." By that time, I was amused by this. He was bringing information to the "expert." I'm telling him I don't understand it, and he keeps talking with me about it. It became clear after several of these visits that simply discussing this research together was therapeutic for him, regardless of whether I had a sophisticated understanding of it or not. My interest and willingness to learn—from him, from others—was what was important. It's been a great lesson for me. I've come to see that patients don't think you have to

know it all to trust you.

Is There Such a Thing as too Much Equality?

The mutual participation model of doctor-patient interaction also has some drawbacks. Throughout the history of medicine, when specific treatments were unknown, much of the "medical magic" or healing power of the physician derived from the patient's faith in this power. Particularly when patients are very ill, the mystique of the physician can be tremendously reassuring and can promote healing by all the unknown means that cause a placebo to work.

Thus, cure of disease may or may not occur, but the healer of sickness (physician, shaman, curandero) must be accepted as having a special and unequal status. As one HIV specialist observed, "When we all become equal, something is gone. I think health does benefit from some ritual, some belief system, based on the authority of the healer. I think that explains why a lot of practices in other cultures do work to promote health, even though they may have no scientific validity."

In addition, responsibilities are always accompanied by burdens. These can be overwhelming, especially for the patient who is experiencing acute medical distress, pain, or fatigue. Some patients may not want to have to think about different treatment options, but would rather just do whatever the doctor thinks is best. A recent front page article in *The New York Times* commented on the new dilemmas faced by patients:

> "We have created a climate which says that the good patient is the most consumer-oriented, who gets the most information and makes the most informed decision," said Dr. Jimmie Holland, Chief of Psychiatry at Memorial Sloan–Kettering Cancer Center in New York. "Patients feel a tremendous obligation to make judgments themselves." Dr. Holland says her staff is frequently consulted by distraught patients who just can't make up their minds. Doctors see their role as helping patients make choices—providing data and lending an informed ear—but many medical ethicists who believe in patient choice say that merely providing patients with large volumes of information—what they call "truth-dumping"—leaves patients not better informed but just confused. (Rosenthal, 1994, p A1).

The burden of having to make critical treatment decisions is distressing and has led some HIV patients to seek counselors for help with this process. Counseling is aimed at alleviating the anxiety and frustrations patients may feel, helping them formulate questions and concerns for the physician, and evaluating the pros and cons of various options.

A more prosaic problem with the notion of equality in the doctor-patient relationship has to do with time: It takes the physician longer to explain treatments, to listen to questions, and to discuss the risks and benefits of interventions. Reimbursement for a routine office visit is granted at a flat rate, regardless of the duration of the visit. In these days of managed care, lower rates are paid to providers who belong to HMOs or who accept Medicare or Medicaid patients. According to one physician, "This is only financially feasible in a high-volume, rapid turnover, efficient, procedure-oriented practice, which does not promote extensive conversation with patients. Everyone wants this fantastic relationship, this ideal relationship with their physician for this very complex disease, but the physician gets paid less." Although HIV specialists do not choose the field for its profit margin, they need to employ considerable office staff to manage the unusual volume of paperwork; they also need to remain solvent if they wish to maintain themselves, their families, and their practices.

EFFECTS OF PROGRESSIVE ILLNESS

The doctor-patient 'partnership' usually changes over time as illness progresses. Under ideal circumstances, the alliance remains even when equality does not.

The Early Stage

Initially, when healthy, the more assertive HIV-positive person is likely to consider his or her physician a consultant or advisor, helping to determine the treatment plan. The patient may even consult more than one physician as part of the process: "At first, I was shopping for a consultant. The decisions had to be mine. It's my body, my life. They [physicians] give me their assessment of the situation; they give me the options as they see them; they recommend what they feel is best, and ask me what I want to do. That's how I like and need and want my care to be handled."

The alert patient is also likely to switch doctors if the first one fails to communicate hope. This is not an uncommon experience, especially if a non-AIDS specialist is the first to be consulted. One patient observed, "I ended up leaving my first doctor because she was basically a grave digger. She said to me on more than one occasion, 'You have a fatal disease and you are going to die,' and not for one second did I accept that as a possibility."

A young woman went to a doctor after testing positive for HIV. She tells the following story:

> He said at my first visit, "The good news is that you don't have any opportunistic infections. The bad news is that you're a walking time bomb. Your T cells are so low, it's only a matter of time before you get sick. You have to be on AZT, you have to be on everything." And when I left his office I was totally flipped out. It was rough. I finally found the doctor [an experienced AIDS specialist] I see now, who I really like. He said, "I'm of the school of thought that maybe this can be a manageable chronic illness." And it was a ray of hope for me.

The Middle Phase

At some point, symptoms begin to appear and prophylactic and acute treatments are needed. As a rule, during this phase, experienced physicians have clear ideas about what they consider appropriate treatment and when it should be initiated, although in the practice of HIV medicine, there is considerable diversity of opinion. In this middle phase, then, doctors usually make clear recommendations and try to persuade patients to agree with them. Patients may also have definite opinions, and during this time, may actively participate in the decision making. When an acute episode ends, the relationship may revert from the guidance-cooperation model to the mutual participation model.

At this time, patients may begin to think about the dual nature of their needs—for healing as well as curing. As one woman observed, "There's more to medical care than giving someone medicine. I think care is about caring and about treating people with respect and dignity and providing them with what they need. I think it's a little more than just dispensing medicine."

As time passes, the relative length of periods of health and illness begin to change. For people diagnosed early in the disease spectrum, there may be an extended period of health with little or no illness. Eventually, however, people begin to experience periods of illness, with clear-cut but progressively shorter intervals of good health. At some point, the balance changes, and illness predominates.

Later Stages of Illness

In later stages of HIV illness, treatment issues often become more complex. Although there is an increasing number of treatments for AIDS-defining opportunistic infections, there eventually comes a point when the established treatments have been tried and no longer work. For example, one man who was first diagnosed with PCP (*Pneumocystis carinii* pneumonia) in 1986 initially recovered completely. In 1989, he developed CMV (cytomegalovirus) colitis. Ganciclovir (Cytovene) was started and was effective for a while. When he developed CMV retinitis, ganciclovir was discontinued and foscarnet (Foscavir) was initiated. Ganciclovir was again added to the regimen when the colitis became active. The retinitis progressed. Throughout this time, the patient brought to the physician's attention a number of experimental treatments (e.g., the gp 160 vaccine trial and retinal implants of ganciclovir), which the physician discouraged. When CMV again became active, despite the simultaneous therapy with the only two recognized treatments, the physician, who had previously held strong opinions about the correct treatment to pursue, was much less assertive about his proposals and asked the patient on several occasions what *he* thought should be done next. For his part, the patient was becoming physically debilitated and emotionally drained. For the first time, he wanted the physician to take charge. He no longer was interested in the kind of partnership he had initially endorsed, nor was the physician. Unfortunately, neither initiated a conversation about this shift. The patient concluded that the physician was giving up, and losing interest in him; the physician perceived the patient as unwilling to acknowledge the reality that there were no more effective treatments. When treatment options dwindle, the doctor-patient relationship has to change.

Another common scenario in later-stage illness is that the patient is too acutely ill to participate in decision making at all, even if the particular illness episode is not regarded as terminal. If the patient is brought to the emergency room with 105° fever, he or she is probably not going to be able, for example, to discuss whether to consider I.V. pentamidine (Pentam 300) with or without steroids in the management of recurrent PCP. As one patient pointed out, "I always made the decisions about my care. But the first week I was in the hospital I was really out of it for several days. The headaches were so debilitating that I was given Dilaudid injections, and at that point, the physician had to make the executive decisions."

The burden of making decisions about medical care is just one more source of fatigue for patients in a long and tiring illness. As treatment options diminish, as illness progresses to restrict mobility and the activities of ordinary life, and discomfort and pain increase, some people become too tired to want to continue pursuing medical options that have diminishing odds of benefit. Someone has to discuss the ending of life, and what the physician's role is going to be in providing comfort at this time.

At the end, in the best cases, the doctor will not vanish from the hospital room. Even though there may be nothing medically left for him or her to do in terms of cure, there is still great value in the role of healer and patient advocate. The wise physician combines the science of curing with the art of healing and knows when one is called for and the other is not.

One physician said, "One of the most important things I can do for a patient and his loved ones is to make death as peaceful as possible. I remember when I read Camus' *The Plague* in high school. I thought the doctor was really unfeeling; he didn't love his patients; he "just" did the best he could. Now I understand. It's not like I can be a hero and fix everybody, but what I can do is stay. I can be there."

At the end, the physician's role as healer becomes paramount. He or she is the ultimate caring figure whose responsibility it is to reassure, to comfort, and to remain steadfast.

REFERENCES
Aoun H. From the eye of the storm, with the eyes of a physician. *Annals of Internal Medicine.* 1992;116:335-338.

Bloom SW. *The Doctor and His Patient.* New York: Russell Sage;1963.

Bloom SW, Wilson R. Patient-practitioner relationships. In Freeman HE, Levine S, Reeder L, et al, eds. *Handbook of Medical Sociology,* 3rd ed. Englewood Cliffs, NJ: Prentice Hall; 1979, pp 275-296.

Cassell E. *The Healer's Art.* Philadelphia: Lippincott; 1976.

Parsons T. *The Social System*. Glencoe, Il: Free Press; 1951.

Rosenthal E. Hardest medical choices shift to patients. *The New York Times*. 1994; January 27:A1.

Rothman D. *Strangers at the Bedside*. New York: Basic Books;1991.

Szasz T, Hollender M. The basic models of the doctor-patient relationship. *Archives of Internal Medicine*. 1956; 97:585-592.

6

TREATMENT STRATEGIES AND PHILOSOPHIES

COMMENT

Expert AIDS physicians hold diverse views and philosophies on treatment. As in other diseases with no proven treatment and no professional consensus, management decisions are often difficult and complex. The advantage, however, is that patients, who also differ in their beliefs about treatment strategies, can usually find experienced physicians whose views match their own.

In light of the limited options available in HIV management, the patient may play a greater role in the decision-making process than in other illnesses. Most physicians work hard themselves at remaining abreast of new developments in AIDS treatment. Thus, while HIV specialists are conservative, for the most part, they are willing to consider new strategies and approaches if some level of efficacy has been established and there is no evidence of harm—or at least no more harm than from available alternatives.

For too many HIV-related conditions, there are no curative treatments, standard procedures, or even widely held beliefs about appropriate management. Consequently, the judgements and personal philosophies of AIDS specialists and of patients strongly influence medical decision making. Major tasks include how to make treatment decisions with little scientific evidence; how to assess the risks and benefits of using a particular treatment at all and whether to initiate such treatment sooner or later; whether and when to try unproven therapies; and how to integrate alternative therapies and conventional medicine.

Both physicians and patients bring particular preconceptions, expectations, and expertise to the task of managing HIV illness. The necessary accommodations and negotiations between physician and patient as part of a mutually trusting and respectful relationship are nowhere more apparent than in their joint attempt to mesh orthodox and unconventional management approaches. Other problems, such as pain and sexual dysfunction, are often present and can raise similarly complicated issues.

This chapter has been expanded with permission from a previously published article in *PAACNOTES* (1993;5:128-132).

MAKING TREATMENT DECISIONS IN THE ABSENCE OF CLEAR EVIDENCE

Most medical procedures and strategies are based on years of clinical experience, without the endorsement of scientific evidence (Smith, 1991). For example, the efficacy of many common medical interventions, such as coronary bypass surgery or ulcer medication, has never been demonstrated in rigorous scientific studies, yet they are widely accepted. While not ideal, clinically based therapeutic regimens are not considered controversial. In less established areas of medicine like HIV illness, however, physicians and informed patients are more likely to turn to the research literature for evidence of the effectiveness of a particular procedure or medication.

The gold standard of evidence in clinical research is the randomized controlled trial. This is, unfortunately, a long-term undertaking. A physician commented in a medical journal editorial, "It takes years for controlled trials to produce the data that physicians and patients need to make rational decisions in the presence of debilitating chronic disease" (Campion, 1992, p 1427). When the endpoint is survival rather than symptom relief, the clinical trial must be extended for years to be meaningful.

Given the newness of most HIV/AIDS treatments, such evidence is largely unavailable. Even the largest, longest, and most extensive trials conducted to date in the United States—the AIDS Clinical Trials Group AZT (zidovudine)/placebo studies—provide limited information because of narrow inclusion criteria; the use of high doses of AZT that are no longer considered necessary for efficacy; and scientifically premature termination on ethical grounds.

One physician offered a classification scheme based on the "state of the evidence" that is helpful in assessing risks, benefits, and certainty in developing treatment strategies for HIV illness. The first category includes treatments that are widely acknowledged as effective; the second consists of antiretrovirals (also widely acknowledged as useful but for a limited time and with additional complications); and the third encompasses unproven, unconventional, experimental, or alternative treatments.

ACCEPTED TREATMENTS

There are, alas, not many "orthodox" treatments for HIV-related conditions. Some do exist, and fortunately the list is growing. There is substantial agreement about the effectiveness of these treatments among physicians and patients, even in the absence of large replicated clinical trials. Evidence of efficacy stems largely from epidemiologic (observational) studies in which large numbers of patients—some of whom have used the treatment in question and others who have not—are followed over time. Differential survival rates, if observed, underscore the value of the intervention being studied. Included in this category are some primary prophylactic treatments (e.g., trimethoprim-sulfamethoxazole [Septra, Bactrim] and DDS [dapsone] for PCP [*Pneumocystis carinii* pneumonia] prophylaxis), some secondary prophylactic treatments (e.g., acyclovir [Zovirax] to prevent recurrent herpes), and some treatments for acute opportunistic infections (e.g., ganciclovir [Cytovene] for CMV [cytomegalovirus] retinitis). Physicians generally agree with each other and with patients on the choice of intervention, timing, and dose for treatments in this category although variations do exist. When the patient's CD4 cell count drops to about 200, for example, most physicians would consider initiating PCP prophylaxis. There may, however, be some variation in dosing: PCP prophylaxis may be prescribed at a dose of three double-strength pills per week, while others may prescribe one or even two per day. Some physicians prescribe ganciclovir for acute treatment of CMV 5 days a week, while others prescribe for 7 days, adjusting the dose accordingly.

Patients almost always accept such treatment plans and cooperate in their implementation. There is little disagreement, for example, about the use of acyclovir for herpes, as both acute treatment and, if recurrent, prophylaxis. Fluconazole has rapidly become the standard treatment for cryptococcal meningitis, and as prophylaxis against recurrences, since its approval in this country. And since its approval in 1993 as prophylaxis for *Mycobacterium* complex (when CD4 cell counts drop below 100), rifabutin (Mycobutin) has been used more frequently, at least by some HIV specialists. In short, a few treatments and interventions are recognized as conventional and even standard in the management of HIV-related conditions.

ANTIRETROVIRAL DRUGS

The antiretroviral class of drugs consists of AZT, ddI (Videx), ddC (Hivid), and d4T (Zerit), which are marketed, and 3TC, which, in 1994, is still classified as investigational. Since some benefit of AZT over placebo (at least in the short run) was already established by the time the ddI and ddC studies were begun, these trials compared the new drugs with AZT and not with a placebo. Although both ddI and ddC are approved by the FDA, they are almost never considered first-line antiretroviral therapy. Thus, for the purposes of this discussion, AZT will be considered representative of the antiretroviral class of medications.

Community Attitudes About Antiretrovirals

Use of AZT, and antiretrovirals in general, is probably more controversial than is any other aspect of HIV management. Since its approval in 1987 as the first compound with any demonstrable therapeutic value in the management of HIV illness, patients have been dramatically divided in their appraisal of AZT. From the outset, some activists sought to increase patient access while others categorically rejected its use. Some opponents, like Michael Callen (Callen, 1990), have been sophisticated and articulate, while others adamantly refuse the medication because "My buddy Joe took it and he died; he was on AZT you know."

Although some of the original antipathy stemmed from the severe anemia associated with the early doses, which were higher than they are at present, this is no longer common. Nevertheless, there is still considerable reluctance among a sizeable number of patients to consider antiretroviral treatment, despite the lack of other treatments available for the HIV illness itself.

Physician Attitudes About Antiretrovirals

Nearly all physicians believe that antiretroviral drugs have a part to play at some point during HIV illness, although identifying that point has become a subject of considerable controversy. Clinical trials have shown that AZT appears to postpone the onset of AIDS, if not the overall duration of survival. AZT may also have a protective role against dementia. In a conservative assessment of efficacy, there appears to be at least a 6- to 18-month period during which the T-cell counts of many patients on AZT either rise or fail to decline, compared with those of patients taking placebo (Fischl et al, 1990).

Many critical questions remain. As noted in a 1994 *New England Journal of Medicine* editorial, "No consensus has been reached about the use of antiretroviral agents throughout the course of HIV infection, principally because the agents currently available are only incomplete inhibitors of viral replication in vivo" (Saag, 1994, p 706).

MANAGEMENT ISSUES: DECISIONS, DECISIONS, DECISIONS

The risks of AZT are both physiologic and psychological. Drug toxicity appears to be dose-related. The major studies, conducted during the late 1980s, used a daily dose of 1200 mg, which is now almost universally considered unnecessarily high. The current recommended regimen for AZT is 600 mg daily in three divided doses; lower doses might be used if another antiretroviral (ddI or ddC) is given concomitantly. At these lower doses, anemia and other toxic reactions are much less common. Possibly transient but nonetheless annoying side effects, such as headache, nausea, insomnia, and muscular pain, may also occur at lower doses.

Some patients appear to become drug resistant after about 6 to 18 months of treatment with AZT. It seems that time to development of resistance may be related to stage of disease when AZT is initiated. More advanced patients tend to develop resistance more rapidly. Such resistance has sparked a debate about when to begin its use. Some physicians argue that if AZT will be effective only for a limited time, it should be reserved for that stage of symptomatic illness when it is really needed (Hamilton et al, 1992). Others, however, argue that protecting the immune system before it deteriorates is most important (Corey and Fleming, 1992).

In an editorial about what to do when AZT fails, the author, a physician, concluded:

> The essential factors to be considered in planning treatment are the demonstrated but limited efficacy of zidovudine [AZT] in retarding the progression of disease and the likelihood that additional antiviral agents will become available for use in the future. If one believes that there will not soon be additional active agents, it is logical to delay antiretroviral

therapy until more symptoms of infection develop. Conversely, if one believes that additional drugs are around the corner, then it makes sense to treat patients earlier in order to delay destruction of the immune system and its consequences (Saag, 1994, p 706).

Treatment with AZT also carries a psychological risk: for nearly all individuals with HIV infection, this is the first "chronic" medication. . . and one that is widely regarded as a clear marker of illness progression. The person is converted into a "patient" with all that that implies. Swallowing the distinctively colored AZT capsules three times a day is a constant reminder of "patient" status.

While almost all physicians recommend the use of antiretrovirals at some point during the course of illness for at least some patients, there is considerable disagreement about when to start treatment, and, to a much lesser extent, about dose. In 1990, a "State-of-the-Art Conference on Azidothymidine [AZT] Therapy for Early HIV Infection," sponsored by the National Institute of Allergy and Infectious Diseases (NIAID), issued the following specific recommendation: "Therapy with zidovudine [AZT] is recommended for both symptomatic and asymptomatic HIV-infected individuals whose CD4 counts are fewer than 500 [optimally done twice at least a week apart]" (NIAID, 1990, p 339).

These guidelines were revised based on subsequent data from large clinical trials. In December 1993, another such "state-of-the-art" conference issued more conservative recommendations regarding AZT (Sande et al, 1993). The new guidelines state that when the CD4 cell count falls to between 200 and 500, either of two options are recommended: 1) initiate AZT treatment at 600 mg/day, or 2) "continue observation with clinical and immunologic monitoring for disease progression, without initiation of antiretroviral therapy" (Sande et al, 1993, p 2584). AZT would then be initiated upon evidence of disease progression, such as rapid decline in CD4 count or the onset of HIV symptoms like persistent fevers, weight loss, or unexplained diarrhea. According to the 1993 guidelines, antiretroviral therapy is recommended for all patients with CD4 cell counts under 200, regardless of the presence or absence of symptoms.

In an interesting departure from the earlier guidelines, the current recommendations explicitly state the importance "of patient involvement in the choice of treatment strategies. Patients and physicians must be aware of the benefits, toxic effects, limitations, and unknowns of the antiretroviral drugs when making treatment decisions. Physicians are obliged to educate patients about clinically sound treatment options and their impact on quality of life.... Accordingly, the current recommendations are less prescriptive than those from a previous state-of-the-art conference held in 1990" (Sande et al, 1993, p 2583).

The prevailing approach among HIV specialists in deciding when to start antiretroviral treatment is to focus on patterns of laboratory indicators, looking for changes over time. The indicators they use and their interpretations, however, are not uniform. The effect of such variations in practice for some patients can mean delayed treatment. For the most part, these physicians have established ongoing relationships with their patients, who are generally reliable and can accurately report their symptoms. For other patient populations, where a long-term physician-patient relationship is either impossible or unlikely, following current guidelines about antiretroviral therapy may be the most reasonable course of action.

UNAPPROVED MEDICAL TREATMENTS

The number of medical procedures and treatments considered to be alternative or unconventional is vast. We, therefore, divide this area into two broad categories: unapproved medical treatments that are nevertheless within the scope of conventional medical tradition and unconventional treatments and procedures that derive from other traditions.

Unapproved medical treatments, are, almost by definition, not supported by conventional scientific evidence. There are at least three kinds of unapproved medical treatments: 1) "off-label" use of marketed medications prescribed for unapproved indications by physicians (e.g., acyclovir for CMV prophylaxis, pentoxifylline [Trental] as an antiretroviral); 2) medical procedures that are approved only for non-HIV conditions if at all and that are available from only one or a handful of investigators (e.g., hyperthermia, passive immunotherapy); or 3) experimental or investigational compounds that are currently in preliminary trials or are approved in other countries but are not available in the United States.

Due to the chronicity and intractability of HIV-related conditions, unproven medical treatments have assumed particular significance and complexity for PWAs (persons with AIDS). In his review of alternative therapies, Abrams observed, "Baffled by the continued lack of effective therapies, [many in the gay community] started an alternative treatment movement that has grown to the point at which most practicing providers caring for patients with HIV infection are likely to have interacted with patients who have chosen alternative therapies" (Abrams, 1992, p 111). There are several biweekly or monthly publications that provide information and updates on AIDS treatment, and Project Inform in San Francisco maintains a 24-hour hotline plus a monthly newsletter that provides information about alternative treatments including unapproved medications and unconventional therapies.

As with most other consumer-driven items, styles and preferences for unapproved treatments change over time. In the early days of the AIDS epidemic, for example, before *any* compound was approved for treating HIV-related illnesses, popular alternative treatments were AL-721 (active lipids in a ratio of 7 to 2 to 1), ribavirin, and inosine pranobex (Isoprinosine). As Abrams observed, "In 1985, studies of Isoprinosine and ribavirin were launched in a number of medical centers. Soon it became known that these same agents were widely available through over-the-counter sales in Mexican pharmacies. Individuals began to cross the border to obtain their own supplies. Occasional skirmishes were reported between border agents and infected importers with their contraband of hope, stories reminiscent of the Laetrile saga of decades past" (Abrams, 1992, p 113).

In 1987, dextran sulfate, obtained from Japan, became a popular alternative treatment. Its increasing availability on the street threatened to interfere with interpretation of data from clinical trials. In response to the controversy surrounding access to and importation of dextran sulfate, the Food and Drug Administration (FDA) announced a new policy permitting individuals to import drugs from foreign countries for personal use under the direction of a monitoring physician. This led Abrams to comment, "The alternative therapies movement had affected the FDA regulatory system for the first, but certainly not the last, time" (Abrams, 1992, p 114).

Although antiretroviral and then other medications were approved for patients with HIV illness beginning in the late 1980s, there is still no cure for AIDS, and unapproved medical therapies have remained popular. In the 1990s, the trendy alternative treatments include, among others, Compound Q (used mostly on the West Coast and believed to have antiretroviral activity), naltrexone (Trexan) (a narcotic antagonist believed to bolster the immune system), and pentoxifylline (Trental) (approved for treatment of occlusive arterial disease and thought by some to have antiretroviral action by reducing tumor necrosis factor serum levels).

Off-Label Use: Using Approved Drugs in New Ways

Most AIDS specialists learn from each other or from their patients about new indications for marketed medications before formal findings are published or approved by the FDA. For example, in the early 1990s, it had been proposed that high doses of acyclovir (up to 4000 mg/day), marketed for the treatment of genital herpes, may constitute effective prophylaxis against CMV. Many specialists had, in fact, tried using acyclovir this way and most no longer use it. "I have done that and it doesn't do a thing. And they may get resistant herpes," one physician explained. Another physician, however, prescribed acyclovir for severely immunosuppressed patients because he believes the chances of CMV outweigh the risks of drug side effects. And another said he didn't think it worked, but he complied with patient requests because he didn't think it would do any harm. Subsequent evidence from a collaborative European-Australian study eventually supported their clinical observations about lack of efficacy for the prevention of CMV retinitis (Youle, 1993).

Most HIV specialists have access to both formal and informal information networks and generally hear about new medical indications early in their development. Unless there are either theoretic or practical reasons to believe that risks will outweigh benefits, they are willing to try an alternative treatment if a patient so requests. These physicians will try something new with several patients and stop if the results are not apparent.

Approved Medical Procedures Used in New Ways

Some medical procedures developed for other purposes have been used either to bolster the immune system or to treat specific HIV-related conditions. Passive immunotherapy, for example, was developed to provide temporary immunity when vaccines for active immunization are unavailable or have not been given before exposure to infection. Passive immunotherapy is accepted treatment for conditions such as rabies, tetanus, and hepatitis B. In the context of AIDS, plasma is taken from HIV-positive asymptomatic donors with high levels of anti-HIV antibodies. The plasma is processed to inactivate HIV and then infused in the recipient who typically has late-stage HIV illness. Several studies conducted in the United States and England have not found this costly procedure to be clinically effective, although adverse reactions have not been noted.

Plasmapheresis (plasma exchange) is procedurally similar to kidney dialysis in that blood is removed from the patient, is filtered through a blood cell separator to remove the targeted pathogen, and is replaced by an equal volume of replacement solution (usually normal plasma along with the patient's red blood cells). The procedure has been found helpful in several disorders, such as myasthenia gravis and Guillain-Barré syndrome. It is, however, costly and possibly hazardous and requires repeated administrations. Plasmapheresis has been proposed by some HIV specialists as a treatment for chronic inflammatory neuropathy, with mixed results reported in uncontrolled case series and trials. For immunosuppressed patients, the added risk of catheter infection is nontrivial.

Another medically legitimate procedure—with very limited indications—that is not approved for treatment of HIV-related conditions is hyperthermia, a technique in which blood is removed from the body and circulated through a special machine where it is heated and then returned. Hyperthermia has been used in cancer treatment, albeit uncommonly, since cancer cells are susceptible to destruction at temperatures of 105.8 °F while normal body cells are not.

In 1990 an Atlanta physician reported rapid and dramatic improvement in KS (Kaposi's sarcoma) lesions, as well as a tenfold increase in CD4 cells, in a patient treated with hyperthermia. After much media attention, enthusiasm for the procedure subsided. Theoretically, hyperthermia seems fairly implausible as a treatment for immunosuppression, since very ill AIDS patients sometimes run fevers of 106 °F or more for a few hours. These very high fevers, however, have not seemed to positively affect AIDS. Moreover, there have been no demonstrated efficacy trials. In addition, we now know that most HIV replication occurs in the lymph system, not the blood. Nevertheless, in 1994, some centers for alternative therapies continue to encourage their clients to go to Rome or Switzerland for this treatment.

While procedures in this category have medical justification in contexts other than AIDS, they may be associated with significant medical risks, as well as high (as a rule nonreimbursable) costs with no clear evidence of efficacy.

Experimental Medical Treatments

This category includes drugs in early clinical trials, often identified by numbers instead of names and accessible only to research participants or those eligible under compassionate-use INDs,* vaccines, and compounds in later stages of research that are not yet approved for marketing in the United States although they may be in other countries. A sharp distinction should not be made among these subgroups since successful drugs can move from one level of study and acceptance to the next fairly rapidly. In the era of HIV disease, "unapproved treatment" is a term also used for "alternative treatment" in the acquisition of medicines from sources like buyers' clubs that sell imported compounds marketed abroad and other drugs that are still in clinical trials with restrictive entry criteria. Medications like clarithromycin (Biaxin), available earlier in Europe, are now marketed in the United States. Before FDA approval, such drugs had been available through American buyers' clubs that imported the drug in bulk and sold it at cost.

While some physicians favor novel treatments in principle, others oppose them, also in principle. The former attitude is illustrated by the physician who explained:

> I think I was always willing to do something different because whatever was available wasn't satisfactory. So I monitored Isoprinosine; I did naltrexone; I did Antabuse, ribavirin. I would send people to wherever I thought they could travel. I was the first one to do passive immunotherapy here in New York. After hearing about that guy in Atlanta who was heating blood, hyperthermia, I had nine KS patients come in the next day. I did skin biopsies and sent them overnight to this guy. I was always looking for some kind of magical something. Now I don't push Antabuse, I don't push cimetidine, I don't push NAC, St. John's Wort. Some patients ask, "What do you think of this?" I used to say, "I tried it, and it didn't do anything. But it's not going to hurt." Now I'm not as eager to give people unproven nontoxic therapies that I have already used and that haven't worked.

This physician is known for a willingness to experiment with novel therapies, and is sought out by patients interested in trying them.

The moderates in this area are the physicians who do not themselves obtain and use experimental therapies but who help patients participate in compassionate trials if usual treatments have failed or if there are no "usual" treatments. Physicians in this category are often willing to recommend unproven treatments as long as at least some evidence (not including anecdotal reports) shows the potential for benefit.

---

*Compassionate-use IND (Investigational New Drug): The FDA can approve an investigational drug for clinical use in a specific patient who is ineligible for research participation and for whom another effective treatment is not available.

The prevailing view among experienced HIV physicians was summed up: "It seems that there is an endless stream of new drugs. For 11 years now, the excitement of unproven new drugs tends to be inversely proportional to what we know about them. I tend to be very skeptical. On the other hand, I consider myself up-to-date and am delighted to provide patients with interventions that I think are likely to be helpful [where evidence already exists]."

At the other extreme are the conservative physicians who, in principle and from a public health perspective, are pleased about trials of new therapies but who advise their own patients not to be guinea pigs, subject to the unknown risks as well as uncertain benefits of unproven therapies.

UNCONVENTIONAL THERAPIES

Even the definition of the term unconventional is controversial, and its borders are permeable. A recent survey about unconventional medicine asked a random sample of American adults whether they had used any of 16 unconventional therapies, defined as "interventions neither taught widely in American medical schools nor generally available in American hospitals" (Eisenberg et al, 1993, p 246). The list included physical therapies like chiropractic, nutritional therapies (e.g., lifestyle diets, commercial weight-loss programs), and a variety of relaxation and "mental" techniques such as spiritual healing, biofeedback, and hypnosis. One in three respondents (34%) reported using at least one unconventional therapy in the past year, and a third of these had seen a provider for unconventional therapy. Extrapolating to the total population, the investigators estimated that Americans made more visits to providers of unconventional therapy than to primary care physicians and spent more money on these visits than is spent annually for all hospitalizations in the United States.

This survey was provocative in more ways than one. Apart from documenting the widespread use and amount of money spent on unconventional therapies, particularly among those with more education and higher income, issues of definition were raised. Indignant readers wrote letters protesting the inclusion of chiropractic as unconventional, asserting "it is conventional, commonplace and appropriate" (Nelson, 1993; Rosener, 1993). Other readers argued against the inclusion of relaxation techniques, acupuncture, herbal medicine, and homeopathy as unconventional.

In a medical journal essay, "Physicians and Healers: Unwitting Partners in Health Care," Murray and Rubel, 1992, proposed four categories of alternative medicine:

- Spiritual and psychological (e.g., faith and spiritual healers, spiritual programs, books and audiotapes, imaging, psychics)
- Nutritional (e.g., specific diets, vitamin and mineral dietary supplements, other supplements like acidophilus, herbal remedies)

- Drugs and biologics (e.g., bitter melon enemas, homeopathy, treatments to enhance the immune system such as urine therapy)
- Treatment with physical forces and devices (e.g., chiropractic, therapeutic massage, acupuncture).

A single practitioner may employ one or several of these strategies.

Jon Greenberg was working on a special edition of GMHC *Treatment Issues* devoted to unconventional therapies just before he died in late 1993. Published posthumously, it was entitled, "An Alternative Treatment Activist Manifesto." He wrote:

> The AIDS community tends to fall into two separate camps regarding alternative therapies. Some dismiss all, regardless of the evidence demonstrating efficacy, and others defend all alternative treatments, regardless of the evidence demonstrating toxicity or lack of efficacy. The reality of most alternative therapies probably lies between these two extremes. Some may be effective, some are clearly ineffective, and most possess some degree of toxicity. They differ substantially in philosophy, modality, cost, and other important ways. However, they all share one unfortunate similarity—virtually nothing is known about their activity in the human body and their efficacy for treating AIDS (Greenberg, 1994, pp 1,2).

Elsewhere he noted that, "…no study of an alternative treatment in AIDS has been able to stand up to scientific scrutiny" because of design flaws, small samples, and other methodologic limitations. He concluded with a plea for well-designed clinical studies of alternative therapies, conducted by the "research establishment," to demonstrate or disprove efficacy.

Cure of the Week: Magic, Folly, and Fraud

All physicians who work with gravely ill patients regularly face questions about "the cure of the week." A magazine published by Project Inform defines "cure of the week" as "mysterious treatments that don't have or invite FDA evaluation or scientific credentials, but which are nevertheless being sold to the public with claims of efficacy" (Tate and Delaney, 1992, p 11). Distinguishing between the truly crazy and the plausible, they point out, is more difficult than it might sound. Nearly all remedies have their proponents, satisfied customers who provide glowing testimonials about the efficacy of the treatment. The desperate patient thinks, "Well, why not me?" While some "alternative therapies" may not be medically effective, they are nontoxic and may promote healing. Others, however, may entail significant risks.

Warning signs of possible quackery include:

1. A specific prohibition against conventional medications or treatments concurrently prescribed. For example, a Hungarian physician working in Switzerland attracted widespread attention in the American HIV community in the early 1990s with his special 18-ingredient herbal mixture, which, he claimed, would boost the immune system and resolve a range of

symptoms from fevers to diarrhea. He required that other treatments, including symptomatic medications like ganciclovir for CMV retinitis, be discontinued to be eligible for his treatment. Moreover, the mixture was expensive, difficult to obtain, and available only from him (GMHC, 1991).

2. Exorbitant cost without explanation for a treatment that is not undergoing serious scientific study. Such treatments may involve extended visits to clinics that require expensive stays of several weeks.

3. Any treatment that claims to cure multiple diseases, especially both AIDS and cancer. Urine therapy, for example, is reputed to "cure any illness, from a common cold to terminal cancer" (O'Quinn, 1980) and has become popular among some PWAs who refer to the treatment as "healing waters" or "auto-urine therapy" (Palladino, 1991).

4. Anybody claiming an HIV cure but whose training is not appropriate or reasonable in the AIDS setting. For example, some AIDS patients have sought out treatment consisting of injections of typhoid vaccine, provided by a nonphysician trained as a syphilologist, who insists all other medications, including PCP prophylaxis, must be stopped. Not only is there no scientific evidence of efficacy, but, as noted in GMHC *Treatment Issues*, "There is a strong theoretical argument for declining this kind of therapy: it is a powerful stimulant of the immune system—exactly the kind of stimulation that makes HIV flourish" (Gingell, 1991).

5. Any remedy that is supported by appeal to a conspiracy theory to explain why it is not more widely known and used. For example, "The government doesn't want people to know about this treatment because it is employing genocidal tactics against AIDS communities." Kemron, an oral form of alpha-interferon given in doses 100,000 times smaller than conventional subcutaneous doses, was claimed in a report from Kenya to dramatically improve patients with HIV, even resulting in some seroreversions (becoming HIV negative). However, at least a dozen studies have failed to replicate these findings: "Despite the volume of data which now prove no benefit to Kemron...scurrilous individuals, including some physicians, have continued to sell Kemron at incredible mark-ups to people with HIV" (Gold, 1993). Even more troubling is the continued federal funding of AIDS centers sponsored by the Nation of Islam, where Kemron still continues to be used as the preferred treatment for PWAs ("AIDS work at a Nation of Islam clinic is questioned." *The New York Times*, 1994).

6. Citing evidence only from obscure publications or institutions; treatment that requires travel abroad; secrecy about ingredients; and claims of HIV seroreversion or characterization of a treatment as "foolproof" or "miraculous."

The authors of the Project Inform magazine article concluded, "The saddest and most dangerous thing about cures-of-the-week, however, is not the money they extract from dying people, it's the harm they do to people who could benefit from more mainstream treatments but who let their health run out pursuing fly-by-night cures...People will go on running to

Mexico, Kenya, Bavaria, and shady practitioners all over America, lured by the promise of miracles. And money is the least important thing they lose" (Tate and Delaney, 1992, p 13).

Placebo Effect

Defining the placebo effect has occupied the attention of scholars for many years. The word itself is a Latin derivation meaning "I shall please." A well-known investigator of the placebo effect defined placebo as "a substance or procedure that is without specific activity for the condition being evaluated" (Shapiro and Morris, 1978, p 371). In research studies, placebos are routinely included for some participants or for some period of the treatment for comparison and to rule out the therapeutic effects of nonspecific elements. For example, if the study involves medication, the placebo is a sugar pill. If the study entails a form of structured psychotherapy, the placebo may simply be sympathetic attention, in the absence of specific therapeutic techniques, for an equivalent number of sessions.

Historically, most treatments offered by physicians have exerted whatever activity they had via the placebo effect. This is probably still true in much of the contemporary nonindustrial world. Positive effects of placebo treatment, which can be potent, have been recorded for disorders as diverse as clinical depression, pain syndromes, hypertension, gastric motility, and dermatitis (White et al, 1978, p 371). Improvement may be due to spontaneous recovery over time, the expectation of improvement and communication of hope instilled by the practitioner, attention given to the patient as part of the treatment, or the treatment act itself (e.g., pill-taking). In general, it should be understood that placebo or nonspecific effects of treatments can occur and can be real.

"New Age Guilt"

One of the unintended consequences associated with the notions of self-empowerment and self-healing is the sense of responsibility when one becomes ill. One patient said, "One of the hardest things for me to work through is the idea that we can control disease by changing our attitudes and lifestyles. I felt like I had failed because I got sick. It isn't just a matter of pulling yourself up with an iron bootstrap. We can't really heal ourselves. In the last analysis, there's a randomness in sickness, a grace in healing."

The notion that disease can be prevented or cured through nutrition, stress reduction, exercise, and other behavioral changes that sometimes fall within the realm of unconventional treatments leads some people to conclude that patients are culpable for their illnesses. This has also been referred to as a form of "blaming the victim." This belief demonstrates a lack of understanding or knowledge about healing and usually exacerbates suffering.

Physicians' Views About Unconventional Treatments

We know of no HIV specialist who endorses holistic, nutritional, or homeopathic remedies as sufficient treatment for HIV conditions, at least once the person has become significantly immunosuppressed and/or symptomatic. One physician said mournfully, "I wish they worked. They are so appealing." Others took a broader view, focusing not on their efficacy as medical treatments but on their healing qualities, impact on overall quality of life, and sense of empowerment:

> Things like acupuncture, homeopathic remedies and Chinese herbs usually share the following phenomena. They're usually harmless; they're usually not terribly difficult [to take]; they don't have a lot of side effects; and they usually make patients feel okay. My feeling is that they are of very little real medical value, but I'm delighted if patients want to take part. I look at it a little like religion: I'm not going to knock your faith in your God. If someone wants to believe that an herb is going to make them feel better, fine with me. It allows patients the ability to be self-directing in their care and have some feeling of control.

Another specialist noted, "I really encourage people to find something for themselves that's healing. That may be hanging out in a cafe, or running, or anything else that isn't weird or unhealthy. I start to object when I see them coming home with two shopping bags of vitamins and believing that 'the more pills I put in my body the better I'll be.' That's what I keep an eye out for and discourage." Similarly, another physician said, "After being much opposed to [holistic approaches] from my traditional background, I am more interested lately. It's the whole idea of empowerment, taking charge. But patients who wish to try nontraditional remedies have got to make the commitment to me as a partner, that they will not alter their monitoring, that they will not go off their conventional drugs, and that they will not drop PCP prophylaxis; that is not negotiable."

A number of specialists are themselves interested in learning more about nutritional interventions and programs. "My new goal in life is to learn more about nutrition because I don't really know anything about it. We were never trained in that stuff. But the whole idea of nutrition being an important component of care is becoming more interesting to me." Indeed, as gastrointestinal diseases and associated malnutrition become more prevalent among HIV-positive patients, the field of nutrition seems to be moving into mainstream medicine. More attention is being paid to maintaining lean body mass from the outset, rather than waiting to intervene until wasting has begun. For example, in the fall of 1993, the cover story of *PAACNOTES* was "HIV and Nutrition". And in December 1993, a major article in *HIV Advances in Research and Therapy* was entitled, "Clinical update: HIV-associated wasting: malnutrition and AIDS progression" (Kotler, 1993).

A "script" was provided by a specialist who suggested the following approach to patients' questions about holistic remedies:

> There's a lot we don't know about many things, and there's a lot I don't know about alternative forms of medicine. That doesn't mean I think

they're either right or wrong. But a lot of alternative forms of medicine do not have the advantage of having been studied systematically. As I see it, my job is to let you know if I think, based on the knowledge that I have, that there is something for your particular situation that you're really making a mistake by not doing, or something I really think you're making a mistake by doing. Anything in between is fair game. But any time anyone suggests that there is only one way to do something or only one approach, you should be skeptical. Patients and their loved ones are often vulnerable because they feel desperate.

Another physician was more succinct: "It's [holistic remedies] okay with me as long as they take the good stuff too." Overall, most HIV specialists are more willing to accept ancillary holistic remedies than many patients think, as long as they remain ancillary.

Although it is difficult to gauge the relative use of conventional and alternative therapies by patients with HIV illness, some evidence suggests that the majority of patients who use unapproved treatments also use conventional medications, at least when their illness progresses to later stages (McCutchan, 1994). It is the rare patient with CD4 cell counts under 200 or 150 who is not on some sort of conventional medications for prophylaxis or treatment of the acute infections that may occur.

While no HIV specialist endorses alternative or holistic remedies as either necessary or sufficient treatment for HIV conditions, if used in conjunction with conventional medications, they are generally considered to have some merit—medically, psychologically, and politically (i.e., the possibility of influencing FDA procedures and regulations). Investigational compounds and approved medications used for new (nonapproved) indications are considered options in the absence or failure of orthodox treatments.

MANAGING PAIN

Inadequate pain management is an oft-repeated criticism of American medical practitioners (Angell, 1982; Solomon et al, 1993; Wanzer et al, 1989; Cleeland et al, 1994). Mild chronic pain, for example, is widespread even among "healthy" people; back pain and other kinds of musculoskeletal and arthritic pain account for high rates of worker absenteeism and social costs (Wells, 1989). Pain is also among the most common complaints of patients using unconventional therapies (Eisenberg, 1993). And fear of uncontrolled pain in terminal illness is a major factor in the public's increasing interest in legalization of physician-assisted suicide (Hamel, 1991).

Pain is a complex phenomenon with physiologic, emotional, and cultural components, none of which is amenable to objective quantification. Willingness to tolerate pain has been a subject of ethical interest since the time of the Greek Stoics, and of religious consideration at least since the days of Augustine. Even in today's secular society, it is often linked to endurance, bravery, and other "machismo" virtues. There is, consequently, a certain social inhibition about confessing to pain and accepting treatment.

Another social barrier to adequate treatment of pain is a reticence by both patients and physicians to use narcotics. Physicians may be professionally concerned about prescribing controlled substances. They may also worry, as do patients, about the perils of addiction, even when the patient is on the deathbed. Even when physicians prescribe analgesics, patients often try to use as little medication as possible, preferring to wait until the pain gets "bad enough." In fact, however, prophylactic use of analgesics to prevent pain onset usually requires less medication than treating existing pain and maintains comfort far more effectively.

Pain Management for Drug Users in Recovery. This is a particularly delicate issue for former drug users and their physicians, both of whom are highly apprehensive about the perils of addiction relapse. As a rule, this occurs rarely, but it is not an entirely unreasonable concern. Special efforts with these patients are appropriate, to ensure adequate tapering of opiates in a safe setting.

Ex-addicts are particularly vulnerable to relapse immediately following a short hospital stay when opiates are prescribed, if not provided with close follow-up. The patient may be reluctant to admit that help is needed. However, the temptation to pick up and use again is great after re-experiencing the physiological and psychological rewards of the drug. As one treatment advocate said, "the body doesn't know if the drug was prescribed or not." If the patient is not kept in the hospital until weaned from the pain medication, follow-up should include making a connection with a substance abuse treatment program. If no formal treatment or substance abuse counselor is available, a friend may fill this role. One woman told about helping a friend who had been prescribed Percocet for pain: "I just went and stayed with her for many days. I brought her to meetings and watched her during that time. I had to insist on doing this because she was afraid to ask for help. But I've seen it happen too often in my community after an acute hospital stay. It's so sad to see someone return to using after 7 or 8 years of sobriety, because sobriety is so valued by us."

Vocabulary. Another significant problem is simply that most physicians and patients lack a pain vocabulary; they fail to distinguish the many types of pain that may be experienced, singly or together. In a survey of over 1,000 oncologists who had cared for 70,000 cancer patients over a period of 6 months, the primary reason given for undertreatment of pain was inadequate pain assessment (Syrjala, 1992). Similar findings were reported in a study of over 1,300 patients with metastatic cancer from 54 treatment facilities. Two-thirds reported significant pain or had used analgesics daily in the past week, and nearly half of these patients were under-medicated (Cleeland et al, 1994). Without the appropriate words to accurately categorize pain, adequate treatment may not be delivered.

THE LANGUAGE OF PAIN

These are some of the words that describe different kinds of pain:

Aching	Throbbing	Exhausting
Shooting	Stabbing	Tiring
Gnawing	Sharp	Penetrating
Tender	Burning	Nagging
Numb	Miserable	Unbearable

To assess pain, one needs to know about:

- Pain duration: fleeting, intermittent, continuous?
- Cyclic patterns?
- What kinds of things ease the pain?
- What makes it worse?
- What medications or treatments have been tried?
- How effective have they been?
- How long does the relief last?
- How troubling are the side effects (if any)?

Finally, if there are several types of pain, and/or several different locations, after describing one site, or one kind, the patient should be asked, or should volunteer information about others that may be present.

Numerous pain management techniques and guidelines have been developed and published over the past 20 years (Cleeland et al, 1994). Despite the fact that "the pain can be controlled by relatively simple means" (Jacox et al, 1994), in as many as 90% of patients, undertreatment continues. New clinical practice guidelines were issued by the federal agency for Health Care Policy and Research in 1994 to address this ongoing problem (Jacox et al, 1994). All too many physicians are less than expert in pain management, and patients, even when they are otherwise informed about HIV-related medical matters, are seldom sophisticated in this area either.

Treatment of pain in HIV illness is particularly important yet often neglected. Pain is widely reported by patients with progressive illness. Breitbart et al (1991) reported in a survey of patients with symptomatic illness attending a specialized PAIN AIDS Clinic at Memorial Sloan-Kettering Cancer Center in New York City that each patient reported an average of three different kinds of pain. While in a few cases, pain may antecede HIV illness (e.g., diabetic neuropathy), it is far more likely to be caused directly by HIV itself (e.g., neuropathies and myelopathies), by KS as it invades soft tissue, by HIV medications (e.g., neuropathic pain associated with ddI and ddC, abdominal pain associated with most antimycobacterial agents), by organomegaly associated with opportunistic infections, or by the direct effects of opportunistic infections (e.g., CMV colitis). It is probably the rare patient with late-stage HIV illness who has not experienced a period of pain, and the lucky patient for whom pain is not chronic.

Treatment for pain may be particularly complicated in the management of AIDS. Physicians tend not to ask about pain or to focus on it, since it is not life-threatening; patients may be reluctant to acknowledge the extent to which pain interferes with their lives. Both patients and physicians may worry unnecessarily about "using up" pain medications when they may need treatment more urgently in the future. In fact, there is no upper limit, no ceiling to the upper-dose ranges of morphine. According to a statement by the Washington State Medical Association (1992), "Using strong opioids earlier during illness does not mean that later on they will be ineffective."

Patients may also be concerned about unacceptable side effects of pain medication—being "stoned," drowsy, or cognitively impaired. There may be gastrointestinal side effects, such as constipation, bloating and nausea, associated with these drugs, as well. Finally, the use of strong opioids may be incorrectly interpreted as an index of approaching death by patients who have seen friends on I.V. morphine in their final illness.

Physician reluctance to address pain may be more easily overcome than patient resistance on this subject. It may be more reasonable, therefore, for physicians to assume this responsibility. Virtually all HIV specialists are familiar with the World Health Organization (WHO) "step approach" to pain management (WHO, 1986). The first step is to recommend nonsteroidal anti-inflammatory drugs (NSAIDs), such as ibuprofen or naproxen, for mild pain. If pain persists or increases, a weak opioid like codeine is substituted, and for moderate pain, oxycodone combined with acetaminophen or equivalent is often prescribed. For severe pain, short-acting or long-acting morphine—oral, liquid, or suppository—may be prescribed, especially if the source of the pain can be identified. For advanced pain, fentanyl (transdermal) patches are often used.

Some HIV specialists pride themselves on their skills in pain management. Nevertheless, this attitude is unusual even among the most experienced HIV specialists. Many can, however, successfully control pain in most instances, in most patients, once that pain has been brought to their attention.

Sometimes pharmacologic problems arise even when patients report pain and physicians prescribe appropriate analgesics. An occasional patient may feel so "drugged" and lethargic that the medicine is considered worse than the pain. In such cases, the physician may lower the dose and add an adjuvant analgesic, try a different medication, or propose an adjunctive trial of dextroamphetamine to offset the lethargy. If that isn't well tolerated, a milder psychostimulant may be helpful. Adjusting both the lethargy-causing medication and its stimulant antagonist requires careful and sustained observation, multiple corrections and adjustments, and patience.

For patients with late-stage HIV illness, the nature of the pain may vary and the location of pain may shift, presenting what often seems like a moving almost elusive target. Moreover, it may take several weeks for an analgesic like morphine to effect maximum pain relief. The patient is also likely to have concurrent medical problems for which he receives additional medications that require adjustment or exchange. Renal or liver impairment, absorption difficulties, and other factors may further complicate the administration and effectiveness of pain medications. While it may be appropriate to refer certain patients to pain specialists for options such as nerve blocks and surgical interventions, people with late-stage HIV illness are seldom eager to involve yet another specialist in their highly complex medical management. This is, however, a worst case and uncommon scenario. In general, satisfactory pain management can be achieved in the context of the primary physician-patient relationship, as long as both partners in that relationship have learned to communicate successfully.

SEXUAL DYSFUNCTION

Sexual dysfunction is a term used to include problems such as low or nonexistent sexual desire, difficulty achieving or maintaining an erection or impotence, and difficulty ejaculating or greatly diminished ejaculate. For women, there may also be problems in lubrication.

Sexual problems appear to be widespread with advancing HIV illness, at least among men. (In this area, as in others, we know of no studies addressing this issue among women.) A significant cause of sexual dysfunction among men is deficient testosterone. Endocrine abnormalities may be a common feature of any late-stage illness (Grinspoon and Belizikian, 1992), and low testosterone is the most frequently identified abnormality in men with HIV. Other causes or contributing factors to sexual dysfunction may include clinical depression, side effects of HIV or psychotropic medications, certain neuropathies involving the groin area, the consequence of systemic illness, or malnutrition induced by metabolic changes

Although sexual activity with a partner may be rare or absent—even in the context of a relationship—as patients become increasingly sick, loss of sexual desire and of interest in masturbation and fantasy nevertheless can be distressing (Rabkin et al, 1993). Sexual dysfunction often becomes noticeable when other manifestations of HIV illness also restrict other enjoyable activities. Sexual dysfunction is one more sign that the patient is losing ground. Lifestyle is changing, becoming more limited. Research on the efficacy of testosterone replacement therapy has shown clear benefit when used to treat hypogonadal men (those with low testosterone).

Treatment is straightforward and can easily be administered in the course of routine medical visits. Many men who are already self-injecting medications themselves can also administer testosterone injections. Yet patients are often reluctant to report sexual dysfunction, and many physicians do not routinely ask. "I wait for the patient to bring it up. I look at testosterone levels only if requested," one physician explained. Another said, "I'll talk about sexual dysfunction if I'm prescribing an antidepressant where it is an expected side effect. Short of that, I tend to wait for the patient to bring it up—which is probably not a good thing. For me, though, it's low on my priority list."

When there are potentially serious medical situations, such as major weight loss, pervasive fatigue, persistent fever, or serious infections, quality of life issues like sexuality indeed tend to be lower priorities. Despite the fact that sexual dysfunction is not life threatening, if both physicians and patients were less reticent, this distressing symptom might be ameliorated.

REFERENCES

Abrams D. Dealing with alternative therapies for HIV. In: Sande M, Volberding P, eds. *The Medical Management of AIDS*, 3rd ed. Philadelphia: Saunders; 1992, pp 111-128.

AIDS work at a Nation of Islam clinic is questioned. *The New York Times*, March 4, 1994, p A18.

Angell M. The quality of mercy. *New England Journal of Medicine*. 1982; 306: 98-99.

Bloom S. *The doctor and his patient*. New York: Russell Sage; 1963.

Breitbart W, Passik S, Bronaugh T, et al. Pain in the ambulatory AIDS patient: prevalence and psychosocial correlates. 38th Annual Meeting of the Academy of Psychosomatic Medicine, Poster Session, October 17-20, 1991.

Callen M. *Surviving AIDS*. New York: Harper Collins; 1990.

Campion EW, Desperate diseases and plasmapheresis (editorial). *New England Journal of Medicine*. 1992;326:1425-1427.

Campion EW. Why unconventional medicine? (editorial) *New England Journal of Medicine*. 1993;328:282-283.

Cleeland C, Gonin R, Hatfield A. et al. Pain and its treatment in outpatients with metastatic cancer. *New England Journal of Medicine*. 1994;330: 592-596.

Corey L, Fleming TR. Treatment of HIV infection—progress in perspective (editorial). *New England Journal of Medicine*. 1992;326:484-486.

Eisenberg DM, Kessler RC, Foster C, Norlock F, Calkins D, Delbanco T. Unconventional medicine in the United States: prevalence, costs, and patterns of use. *New England Journal of Medicine*. 1993;328:246-252.

Fischl MA, Richman DD, Hansen N, et al. The safety and efficacy of zidovudine (AZT) in the treatment of subjects with mildly symptomatic human immunodeficiency virus type 1 (HIV) infection: a double-blind, placebo-controlled trial. *Annals of Internal Medicine*. 1990;112:727-737.

Friedman R, Zuttermeister P, Benson H. Unconventional medicine (letter to editor). *New England Journal of Medicine*. 1993;329:1201.

Gay Men's Health Crisis (GMHC). Swiss therapy still under question

(Treatment briefs). GMHC *Treatment Issues*. 1991;5:10.

Gingell B. Typhoid vaccine therapy (February 1988). In: Armington, K, ed. *GMHC Treatment Issues: Compilation Issue*. New York: Gay Mens Health Crisis; 1991, p 21.

Gold D. Low dose oral alpha interferon ("Kemron"): drug company watch. *GMHC Treatment Issues*. 1993;7:11.

Greenberg J. An alternative treatment activist manifesto. *GMHC Treatment Issues*. 1994;7(special winter 93/94 issue):1-2.

Grinspoon SK, Bilezikian J. HIV disease and the endocrine system. *New England Journal of Medicine*. 1992;327:1360-65.

Hamel R, ed. *Choosing Death: Active Euthanasia, Religion and the Public Debate*. Philadelphia: Trinity Press International; 1991.

Hamilton JD, Hartigan PM, Simberkoff MS, et al. A controlled trial of early versus late treatment with zidovudine in symptomatic human immunodeficiency virus infection—results of the Veterans Affairs Cooperative Study. *New England Journal of Medicine*. 1992;326:437-443.

Jacox A, Carr D, Payne R. New clinical-practice guidelines for the management of pain in patients with cancer. *New England Journal of Medicine* 1994;330:651-55.

Kotler DP. Clinical update: HIV-associated wasting: malnutrition and AIDS progression. *HIV Advances in Research and Therapy*. 1993;3:17-23.

Kotler DP. Pathophysiology of malnutrition. *PAACNOTES*. 1993;5:402-405.

McCutchan JA. Unproven and unconventional therapies. In: Broder S, Merigan T, and Bolognesi D, eds. *Textbook of AIDS Medicine*. Baltimore: Williams and Wilkins; 1994, pp 807-812.

Murray RH, Rubel A. Physicians and healers: unwitting partners in health care. *New England Journal of Medicine*. 1992;326:61-64.

Nelson CF. Unconventional medicine (letter to editor). *New England Journal of Medicine*. 1993;329:1201.

NIAID. State-of-the-art conference on azidothymidine therapy for early HIV infection. *American Journal Medicine*. 1990;89:335-344.

O'Quinn JF. Urine *Therapy: Self Healing Through Intrinsic Medicine*. Fort Pierce Fla: Life Science Institute; 1980.

Palladino Q. Urine therapy: disease carries with it its own cure. *Body Positive*. 1991; 4:8-9.

Parsons T. *The Social System*. Glencoe, Ill: Free Press; 1951.

Rabkin J, Remien R, Katoff L, et al. Resilience in adversity among AIDS longterm survivors. *Hospital and Community Psychiatry*. 1993;44:162-167.

Retrovir's US sales decline. *SCRIP*. 1994;1898:21.

Rosner AL. Unconventional medicine (letter to editor). *New England Journal of Medicine*. 1993;329:1201.

Saag M. What to do when Zidovudine fails (editorial). *New England Journal of Medicine*. 1994;330:706-707.

Sande M, Carpenter C, Cobbs G, et al. Antiretroviral therapy for adult HIV-infected patients: recommendations from a state-of-the-art conference. *New England Journal of Medicine*. 1993;270:2583-2589.

Santosh S. Unconventional medicine (letter to editor). *New England Journal of Medicine*. 1993;329:1202.

Shapiro A, Morris L. The placebo effect in medical and psychological therapies. In: Garfield S, Bergen A, eds. *Handbook of Psychotherapy and Behavior Change*, 2nd ed. New York: John Wiley & Sons; 1978.

Smith R. Where is the wisdom? The poverty of medical evidence. *British Medical Journal*. 1991; 303:798-9.

Solomon MZ, et al. Decisions near the end of life: professional views on life-sustaining treatments. *American Journal of Public Health*. 1993; 83:14-23.

Syrjala KL. Strategies for patient and family support. In *Pain Management and Care of the Terminal Patient*. Seattle: Washington State Medical Association; 1992.

Tate L, Delaney M. Hope, folly or fraud? *PI Perspective*. 992;April:11-13.

Use of antiretroviral drugs in HIV disease declines following preliminary results from Concorde Trial. *Journal of the American Medical Association*. 1994; 271: 488-489.

Wanzer S, Federman D, Adelstein J, et al. The physician's responsibility toward hopelessly ill patients: a second look. *New England Journal of Medicine*. 1989;320:844-849.

Washington State Medical Association. *Pain Management and Care of the Terminal Patient*. Seattle: Washington State Medical Association; 1992.

Wells K, Stewart A, Hays R, et al. The functioning and well-being of depressed patients: results from the Medical Outcomes Study. *Journal of the American Medical Association*. 1989;262:914-919.

White L, Tursky B, Schwartz G. *Placebo: Theory, Research and Mechanisms*. New York: Guilford; 1978.

World Health Organization (WHO). *Cancer Pain Relief*. Geneva:WHO;1986.

Youle M. Double blind placebo-controlled trial of high dose acyclovir for the prevention or cytomegalovirus disease in late-stage HIV disease (abstract MoBoo56). Amsterdam: Eighth International Conference on AIDS; 1992, vol. 1, p Mo15.

LEARNING TO LIVE WITH HIV

COMMENT
*Early in the AIDS epidemic, people discovered their seropositive status
only when they became ill with a life-threatening condition. Today, many
people know they are HIV-positive well before they experience significant
symptoms. The problems associated with this stage of HIV illness—
uncertainty about the future, emotional reactions ranging from disbelief to
acceptance, decisions about disclosing HIV status to others, and adjustments in lifestyle that must be faced—are increasingly common as people
become aware of their seropositive status earlier and earlier in the course of
the infection.*

TESTING POSITIVE

People decide to undergo HIV antibody testing for a variety of reasons. Some,
knowing they are in a high-risk group, find the anxiety of not knowing worse
than the prospect of having their fears confirmed. Others, who believe
they are infected, feel that they might slow or prevent disease progression
with early treatment. Some may seek testing after committing to a monog-
amous relationship, hoping to dispense with "safer sex." Still others seek medical attention for symptoms without being aware that these may indicate the
presence of HIV disease. And sometimes the decision isn't even voluntary.
An emergency hospital admission for an acute, life-threatening opportunistic infection, most often *Pneumocystis carinii* pneumonia (PCP), is
likely to include antibody testing and a diagnosis of AIDS. Similarly, after
childbirth, a mother may be identified as HIV-positive if the baby is ill and
is then tested.

The Early Years

In the early years of the epidemic, before antibody testing became available,
asymptomatic individuals simply did not know they were seropositive,
although some may have had their suspicions. Indirect evidence of HIV
infection, such as a low blood count or even a positive antibody test
obtained in Europe, was difficult to interpret. As one man pointed out, "I was

in a study and our blood samples were sent to Europe, so I found out I was HIV-positive around 1984. It didn't have the emotional impact that perhaps it would today because no one really knew what it meant at the time. It was just another test with a bunch of numbers."

Some people reported that it was a relief to "finally know that all of these bizarre things that were happening to their bodies at least had a name." Some were so acutely ill that the larger implications of the diagnosis weren't considered until later. "It seemed to happen overnight. Suddenly, I woke up breathless and was hospitalized. The first week I was too sick to react, to think. I concentrated on breathing." Another observed, "When I first became sick, I put all my energy into getting better. I would deal with it [the fact of having HIV disease] when I got out of the hospital." Others were indignant: "They said it only happened if you were promiscuous and I was never that. So why me?" More commonly, however, among gay men and drug users, the reaction tended to be, "Why not me?"

In those early years, ignorance was both an asset and a liability. It was not obvious then that nearly everyone who was HIV-positive would probably progress to illness. People were sometimes more upset by the way they were treated in hospitals (e.g., food trays left outside their doors) than by the implications of the diagnosis. On the other hand, those who became ill seldom knew other people with AIDS. Formal and informal resources were meager, and there wasn't any obvious place to turn for information and help.

Changing Circumstances and Attitudes

Attitudes changed in 1987 with the introduction of AZT. Because AZT was thought to delay illness, knowing one's HIV status made sense in terms of protection and prophylaxis. Active treatments were identified, and there was a sense that a cure would be discovered in the foreseeable future. Community groups offering social and financial aid appeared in HIV epicenters. Food for the homebound, foster care for pets during hospital stays, and support groups provided a sense of community support.

As the epidemic continues—and knowledge about the disease grows—discovery of HIV seropositive status can be more unsettling than it had been in the past. Today, a blood analysis performed in conjunction with HIV antibody testing may reveal not only seropositivity but also low T4 cells—currently an AIDS-defining condition. Results such as these indicate that the individual probably has been infected for a long time, and imply there may not be a lot of time left. A low T-cell count in 1986, by contrast, was less alarming because its meaning was largely unknown.

Although it clearly is shocking to receive a diagnosis of AIDS at the time of initial discovery of HIV seropositivity, it is nevertheless also traumatic to receive a positive test result when "asymptomatic." In fact, some individuals who do not have signs of illness consider the term asymptomatic to be misleading. In discussing the effects of being HIV-positive, one person observed, "There is never truly a moment of being asymptomatic with this disease. From the moment a person tests positive, there is something to deal with." Echoing this notion a physician remarked, "There are psychological consequences associated with any illness that lasts longer than 3 days."

STAGES OF RESPONSE

Shocked and Surprised

Many people in the gay and drug-user communities who test positive are not completely surprised. However, as growing numbers of women and their children start to become ill through infection from bisexual or drug-using partners, they are usually completely unprepared for the discovery.

It would seem that people who are members of a high-risk group would be less shocked to learn they are HIV-positive than those who are in low-risk groups. However, it doesn't always happen that way. One woman, who might have realized that certain behaviors put her at risk, said,

> My boyfriend and I got tested because we didn't want to use condoms any-more. He was an I.V. drug user and I had been very promiscuous before that, but I still didn't think there was a snowball's chance in hell I'd come up positive. I just went skipping and hopping into that office to get my [HIV antibody] test results. I knew the technician was going to say, "Your test came out negative." But she didn't say that. I just couldn't believe it. I still can't believe it 2 years later and I don't think I'll ever believe it.

A man who had worked at a major AIDS service agency for many years and who had been told in 1979 that he had GRID (Gay Related Immune Deficiency, a name that preceded AIDS) said, "When I first got PCP in 1986, I practically freaked out. I couldn't get over that I was a dead man. That's all I told anyone who came to visit me. 'I'm a dead man.' I worked here (at the agency) for 7 years, a lot of it doing direct client contact. You can't tell me I'm going to make it after I have seen hundreds of people die."

Regardless of the reasons for seeking HIV testing, receiving a positive result is overwhelming and is often experienced as a death sentence. One man described his feelings this way:

> I can remember the first time I perceived I could be at risk for AIDS. I had never thought I would have to be concerned. I ran, I was young, I wasn't a slut, and I was healthy. But in January 1985, I developed the flu. For 5 days and nights I felt miserable and ran high fevers, so I decided to see a physician. I had recently moved to Boston and did not have my own doctor. So, I went to a local clinic and received a thorough exam. After the exam, the first question the physician asked was, "Are you gay?" I will never forget that moment, and I don't think I will ever experience another like it. As I answered, "Yes," it was as if all the emotions I had ever felt in my life were being poured over the top of me and I could feel them all run from my head to my feet. I was literally numb."

Adjusting to seropositive status is a long-term process that involves questioning assumptions about many aspects of one's life and rethinking priorities and goals. It may even involve a redefinition of self.

The emotional impact of testing positive may include feelings of disbelief, grief and depression, anger, shame and guilt, and, eventually, accommodation. These emotions may not occur in a linear sequence; rather, they may change from moment to moment—a situation that some have described as an emotional roller coaster. Some days patients are able to keep their hands in the air while laughing; other days, all they can do is clutch their hands tightly and scream.

For most people, the initial intense distress usually dissipates after 6 to 8 weeks, and some sense of equilibrium is regained. Researchers at Cornell Medical College (Perry et al, 1993) found that after competent counseling, measures of anxiety and depression assessed 8 weeks after notification of HIV test results returned to pre-test levels for all who participated in the study, regardless of the outcome of their tests.

Disbelief

Disbelief is one of the most common first reactions to receiving a positive HIV test result. One man who had generalized lymphadenopathy and whose test was positive recalled rushing out to investigate all the medical conditions that could produce this symptom. He insisted on having multiple blood tests in an attempt to prove he was not HIV-positive. It took him 2 or 3 months to synthesize this knowledge and incorporate it into his life.

Trying to absorb the news usually takes time, and disbelief is one strategy for creating time. Disbelief allows people to gradually integrate the devastating knowledge of their illness into their lives. If one looks and feels well, it may be particularly difficult to adjust to the notion that one's life will be cut short. While disbelief may be adaptive, it can also keep people from important tasks, including education about HIV and planning for change.

Grief and Depression

Grief and heartbreak are inevitable reactions to the discovery of HIV infection and the accompanying intense sense of loss: the loss of freedom to live each day without the threat of sudden illness, the loss of freedom to make plans for the future and of growing old, the loss of one's health, and the loss of freedom and spontaneity in sexual behavior.

A sense of loss can occur long before physical manifestations of disease begin. And for some, loss of custody or of the potential to have children is devastating. One woman described the loss of her children when her estranged husband discovered that she was HIV-positive in 1986: "At that time everything was so new. He immediately took me to court and got custody of the children. There wasn't a thing I could do." Another said, "Before I was diagnosed, I always had this idea that I'd get married and have children. And then in a second it was all taken away from me, and I felt,

'Well, what is my purpose here in life? What is my legacy? What will I leave behind?'"

Anger

One man told this story:

> I initially had a lot of anger about being HIV-positive. It was mostly directed at a past lover who was sexually compulsive. When we had first met, safer sex was just being talked about, and since neither of us knew much about this or paid much attention to it, we were not using condoms. It was about 2 1/2 years after we had met and started living together that I discovered that my lover had been having multiple sex partners outside of our relationship, and although he said it was always "safe," just the realization that he had not been honest with me about his affairs made me question his ability to be honest about his so-called safe behavior. I had attended a program about self-discovery and freedom and part of this program was a section about anger. As a focus for my anger, I used my past lover and the possibility that he had give me HIV. We were dismissed one at a time from the room by one of the facilitators, and as my facilitator came to me and asked if I was O.K., I just began to sob. I wept for 10 to 15 minutes. I wept because I realized that I was very angry at myself for not having taken better care of myself, and despite my lover's behavior, which I did not like and was still angry about, I was angrier with myself for not being responsible.

Anger is often a major reaction to the discovery that one is HIV-positive. The anger may be directed at possible sources of infection, such as blood banks, past sexual partners, or needle-sharing friends, or it may be directed at oneself for not having been responsible for past behavior. Some feel anger at "God" for the "injustice" of being infected before anything was known about the virus or protection against it. In addition to anger, there may be a feeling of impotence in the face of a disease with no cure. And there is a sense of helplessness and frustration when friends and family members die. There may also be anger at the medical and political establishments for what is often perceived as their feeble response to the AIDS epidemic.

Anger can be energizing, providing the impetus for AIDS activism, such as ACT-UP, and may contribute to improved health. In fact, among long-term survivors, the predominant emotion is not sadness or anxiety, but anger (Rabkin et al, 1993). Anger is often linked to the "fighting spirit" that some people with AIDS consider the explanation for their continued psychological and physical survival. If anger is misdirected and unfocused, however, it may alienate others, including those who want to be supportive. It may also interfere with accomplishing necessary tasks and moving forward productively.

Shame and Guilt

The notion that HIV infection is a punishment for sin (drug addiction, sex between men, sex in general) has become the war cry of many religious fundamentalists, regardless of doctrine. Homosexuals who have not come to terms with their sexual orientation before diagnosis may react to the knowledge of HIV seropositivity with guilt and intensified internalized homophobia. This response is probably extremely rare, however, at least in larger cities among men who are openly gay. More common is the sense of shame, of being "damaged goods," that others would naturally shun, especially in terms of intimacy and sexuality. Some gay men have described feeling "contaminated" and "dirty," foreswearing all future sexual encounters because of negative self-images and the perception of being tainted.

A 29-year-old upper-middle-class woman who worked in the fashion industry discovered to her amazement that she was HIV-positive: "I had the same prejudices that a lot of other people still have about the disease. I thought everybody's going to think I'm a slut. Nobody's going to believe I'm not a drug addict. I was really, really ashamed about being HIV-positive for a long time."

Sometimes these feelings are induced or magnified by the reactions of others. A 45-year-old woman with a long history of drug abuse and prostitution succeeded in turning her life around after learning that she was HIV-positive. However, when she started working at a residential treatment center for addicts, she discovered that,

> The other people who worked there sat around in the staff office talking about disgusting AIDS people. These are people they're supposed to be caring for, and the taxpayers are trusting them, right? It's a fraud, giving millions of dollars to workers who consider the people they are supposed to rehabilitate as less than garbage. That was so traumatic.... the things they said about people with AIDS. I said to myself, "I ain't never going to tell anybody that I have this disease." I just felt terrible about myself as a person.

Another more recent source of shame is having to acknowledge to parents and friends that, in spite of all that is known about HIV transmission, one was careless enough to be recently infected. This feeling is particularly prevalent among very young men who are mortified by the prospect of having to tell their parents how irresponsible they have been. One young law student sought psychiatric treatment specifically because he was so distraught about having to confess his carelessness to his parents, not because of anxiety about future illness or a foreshortened life. Of course, many people who discover their positive HIV status today were infected years ago, before much was known about HIV transmission. Even though they could not have known they were engaging in high-risk behavior, these people may also feel shame and guilt.

Coming to Terms

Learning to live with HIV is a prerequisite to getting on with other goals. Some people claim they have been able to make peace with the virus. One woman described how she bargained with the virus: "Living with this disease sucks, but I decided to make a deal. I said to the virus, 'Look, you're going to live with me until I die, so since I have to live and die with you, let's make a deal. I'll let you rent space in my body and I won't even charge you, but you must be kind to me. I'll try to do the best I can to keep you under control.' And that's what I've been doing ever since."

More often, the process of coming to terms with being HIV-positive is not so explicit. Whether or not acceptance helps people live longer may not matter. It does seem to help people feel they have some control over their situation.

COPING IN THE EARLY STAGES

Adjusting to HIV-positive status while still apparently healthy presents different challenges compared with those faced by those who are clearly sick. In some ways, the problems are more ambiguous and complicated in the early stages. Many questions have no answers: How long will it take for me to get sick? What if I become emaciated and bedbound? Will I be in horrible pain? What can I do or what treatment can I take to stop this from happening? Who will take care of me? How can I maintain hope in the face of such uncertainty?

Life in the early stages of HIV illness is characterized by a sense of overwhelming uncertainty: uncertainty about health, potential for illness, survival, or cure; uncertainty about long-term plans, career goals, and finances. Some described it as a time bomb with a fuse that is becoming shorter and shorter, "Only you can't see the fuse or how much of it is left." One man said: "I kept waiting for the bomb to explode, but it didn't."

In the beginning, the difficulty of accepting HIV-positive status may be compounded by the fact that people look and feel well—in direct contradiction to the generally held notion that "HIV equals death." The uncertainty is confusing. One man explained, "I have often heard it said that we're all going to die at one time or another; you can walk out in the street and be hit by a truck. But living with HIV infection is learning to see the truck coming closer to you each day of your life." Unlike living through the later stages of illness, when the next step is clearer, living through the early stages of HIV challenges people to learn how to achieve balance and perspective in the face of uncertainty—not knowing when the truck will arrive—coupled with the sense that it will inevitably arrive.

Disclosure: Whom and When to Tell

For people who discover they are HIV-positive through an antibody or blood test, there is usually no urgency about disclosure (except to sex- or needle-sharing partners). For those who find out when they are hospitalized for an acute illness such as PCP, however, there is no way to keep the information from the medical and support staff, who may be informed before the patient. Friends and relatives also may find out during hospitalization. Moreover, the life-threatening nature of an initial illness may also involve contact with and disclosure to social workers, lawyers, and clergy.

Disclosure is a highly charged topic for most people. Some react to discovery of seropositivity by isolating themselves and refusing to tell anyone, whereas others respond dramatically and feel they must "tell the world." Neither of these extremes is adaptive. The consequences of total silence are eventually detrimental and burdensome, and it is a barrier to any close relationship. On the other hand, sometimes disclosure can have clearly negative consequences—abandonment by one's partner, loss of insurance, or the withdrawal of so-called friends. In some professions, such as architecture or the performing arts, clients may avoid hiring people known to be HIV-positive for fear that they will not be able to fulfill their commitments. Promotions and job opportunities may be lost. Some of these consequences are due to social stigma and intolerance, whereas others are caused by realistic concerns about endurance and capacity to perform.

People often start the process of disclosure by telling a best friend, sometimes even before they tell a spouse or lover. The way this person responds may influence decisions about other disclosures. Our clinical experience suggests that gay men have more difficulty telling their families than do drug users, and men in general have more trouble than women. There seem to be two sources for this reluctance: the first is fear of rejection and the second is regret about bringing sadness to others' lives.

Men whose parents know they are gay may have a family history of conflict and emotional distance. While past experience may make them more cautious about disclosure, a negative family reaction should not be presumed. One man told us, "At the time I was diagnosed, I had just emerged from an ugly, painful year and a half of not speaking to my father over gay-ness, during which time he aged about 20 years. It really was harder on him than it was on me. And AIDS seemed to have the same effect on him that it had on me. It got us over a lot of silliness. It whittled things down and made it clear we had to work some things out." Another man, who had not told his family anything about his lifestyle or health status, spoke with his sister long-distance after he had been hospitalized twice: "She said, 'What's going on? Is Jimmy your lover? Are you gay? Do you have AIDS?' I said, 'The answer to all those questions is yes.' She said, 'Why haven't you told me? All these years? What did you think I'd do—treat you like a leper? You're like a father to me. You always have been and you think I'm going to treat you like some kind of jerk?' So that was good. And now she refers to Jimmy as her brother-in-law."

A very young man with AIDS who came from a large Catholic family was somewhat removed from his family. When his sister invited him to her wedding, a relative called him to say he shouldn't come because it would spoil the festive mood. His sister, however, said she would not proceed with the wedding ceremony in his absence. He couldn't decide what to do, but eventually his eagerness to attend the celebration outweighed his anxiety about family rejection:

> And I went and people were incredible. Sixty-something-year-old aunts and real religious Catholics, coming right up to me and bringing up the subject themselves. One of my favorite old aunts came up to me and said, "We didn't know you were sick. Such a horrible disease. If you need anything, you know...." They were very moved. And it made a world of difference to my parents. Some of the relatives would say, "Can we do anything for you?" And my response to most of the relatives is, "Stay close to my parents. Drop me a line once in a while, but the best gift I could ask for is knowing that my parents have support."

Even when families do not behave lovingly, their rejection may be a valuable lesson in coming to terms with reality.

> One of the worst things about my diagnosis was seeing people walk out of my life—in particular, my father. My stepmother and I have always been at odds with each other, so I didn't expect that to change, but I saw my father differently than the way he really is. That recognition has been painful, but I've come to accept it and that acceptance has calmed me down and supported me in getting on with my life. It isn't like I wouldn't love his support, but it's not in the cards.

Some people are extremely concerned about the pain their illness will cause loved ones. Others refrain from telling their family out of concern that this will only add to their own burden. One man explained:

> I didn't tell my parents for 2 years after I was diagnosed for a very specific reason. I knew they would fall apart and I would end up having to take care of them. And I was the one who needed to be taken care of at that point. So I didn't need the extra stress of them carrying on and fainting. I waited 2 years so I could say to them, "Look, I'm fine. I've been fine for 2 years and I'm going to remain fine." That worked. They're still very upset but it was a better way and I think I made the right decision.

Parents whose gay sons live in AIDS epicenters such as New York City, Los Angeles, or San Francisco have probably considered, and probably worried about, HIV exposure. Maintaining the secret is an added burden, and barrier, for both child and parents in such cases.

Some people find it easier to inform their parents through intermediaries rather than confront them directly. "I asked my sister to explain it to my parents because I just didn't want to break down and lose control," one man said.

Some men resist disclosing their illness to their families at all costs. They say that they don't want to upset their parents until they are so sick they can't manage alone any more. Or, they feel that their parents are too old or uninformed (especially mothers) to handle the news. If they are the second child in the family to face a foreshortened life, they may be especially concerned about their parents' ability to adjust to disclosure. (A surprising number of men had brothers who also had AIDS, often, but not always, because of the same risk factor.) One man told us, "The hardest part of being diagnosed was telling my mother. She didn't accept it. I had a brother who was bisexual. He died, and his wife died, and their children had it."

A particularly painful task for parents who are HIV-positive is telling their children. One woman said, "I was in jail when I told my 21-year-old daughter. She came to visit me and I said, I'm infected with the virus. I have HIV.' And she said, 'So what? I still love you, that doesn't change anything.' She said, 'I know about it, I read about it, I work with it, so what?' You know, I think that was like the beginning of my life. I was being born again knowing that she was still there, that she understood it."

While some PWAs (persons with AIDS) are rejected or further alienated upon disclosure of their HIV status, more often, they are surprised to discover their parents' supportiveness and affection. In fact, family members are often upset that they were not informed sooner; if they reunite only as the person is dying, their grief is compounded by the anguish of this silence.

OUTING: IDENTIFICATION OF PUBLIC FIGURES

In the early 1990s, some gay activists undertook to reveal the seropositive status of public figures, particularly those considered unsympathetic or indifferent to the needs of people with HIV illness. This became referred to as "outing." In some instances, such as that of Arthur Ashe, knowledge that a newspaper reporter was going to write about his HIV status led to public disclosure, forestalling the revelation by others. Sometimes this has been done posthumously, as in the case of Rock Hudson in 1985 or Rudolph Nureyev in 1993, neither of whom acknowledged their illness while alive. It is certainly helpful for admired public figures to let the world know about their HIV status, and that everyone is vulnerable to the virus. They are praised for going public— "unknowns" do not have a reputation at stake. Public figures who announce their HIV status can contribute significantly toward public education about risk reduction (as in the case of Magic Johnson). This should, however, be a personal decision, not one coerced by outside pressures or threats of disclosure.

Choosing a Physician

The first task to be addressed after discovery of HIV seropositivity is selection of a physician. The antibody test only confirms the presence of antibodies to the virus; laboratory blood tests are required for information about stage of immunosuppression.

Finding a physician is less complicated for people who have HIV-positive friends whom they can ask for recommendations. If a specific physician is recommended often, he or she may be a reasonable place to start. Some people ask their internists for referrals, or call community-based AIDS organizations or AIDS hotlines for names.

Finding a physician with whom one is comfortable, however, isn't always easy. As one woman pointed out, "My HIV-positive friends and I have found that locating a doctor you're comfortable with doesn't usually happen right away. People aren't trained to search for the right doctor; I never expected that I'd have to be a consumer advocate for my own health. I always thought doctors just gave you medication and sent you away, and you got better and that was that. Not that they were human, really, or that you'd want them to be human (laughs)."

From a public health perspective, it is preferable for the family doctor to provide surveillance and treatment early in the course of the illness. In early 1994, Dr. Philip Lee, Assistant Secretary of the Department for Health and Human Services, said in an interview, "Too often, when a patient is found to be infected, the family doctor quickly refers the patient to a specialist or center, often far away, when special treatment is not yet needed. There are simply not enough infectious-disease specialists to care adequately for the growing numbers of people living with HIV." Similarly, Kristine Gebbie, former White House AIDS Policy Coordinator appointed in 1993, said, "Many people can get the care they need closer to home with providers they know" (Leary, 1994, p A21).

Although the need for this public policy perspective is clear, it is also true that a physician who has many other HIV-positive patients, who is experienced, knowledgeable, sympathetic, and interested in treating HIV-related conditions will provide the best care.

Just as no single university is the best for all students, no single physician is clearly the best for all patients. What is more important is the doctor-patient fit or match. Assuming that the doctors being considered are all experienced, knowledgeable, and respected, personal style makes a difference. A female physician observed, "Practices attract people who want a certain type of doctor. Some patients wouldn't like a doctor like me. It would feel too informal, too casual, no white coat, no mirror on the head. They might prefer a more traditional doctor. The informality here, the atmosphere, and maybe having a lot of women around creates an environment that suits some patients better than others."

There are several different styles of practice among HIV specialists. Some are business-like: Their offices run on schedule; brief visits are limited to the time allotted (except if otherwise indicated for strictly medical reasons); and attention is always directed to symptoms, lab results and treatment options. Other physicians are apt to become more personally involved with patients, and may spend extra time providing encouragement and support, or just listening when necessary. The corollary of this "warmer" style is the risk of significant delay for patients in the waiting room; in such offices a wait of an hour or more beyond the specified appointment time is common.

Another important dimension to consider in choosing a physician is treatment philosophy and attitudes about medications, both marketed and experimental. If the patient has strong convictions one way or the other about this, he or she should select a physician who is similarly inclined.

Another essential question concerns finances. What kind of insurance does the physician accept? What is his or her policy toward patients whose private insurance runs out? Is he or she willing at that point to accept Medicaid or Medicare reimbursement? What about uninsured patients?

Education
Education about HIV usually begins when one learns of seropositivity. Some knowledge is acquired during the process of selecting a physician, but a great deal must be learned, and this characteristically takes place over an extended period of time.

Discarding Misconceptions. Even people who consider themselves sophisticated and educated usually harbor some incorrect notions about the transmission, course, and ultimate outcome of HIV infection. Early in the epidemic it was believed—and it is still believed by some people today—that only sexually promiscuous people or I.V. drug users are at risk. A gay man who worked as a volunteer for the Gay Men's Health Crisis Hotline was shocked to discover in 1987 that he had AIDS: "I didn't think the volunteers at the GMHC got it. I know that sounds stupid but really, I never dreamed I'd have it." Debate continues about the magnitude of the risk of infection among the non–drug-using heterosexual population.

The mode of transmission of HIV is still imperfectly understood. In the early years, misconceptions were rampant, and even hospital personnel shunned contact with the ill, leaving their food trays outside hospital rooms, and wearing gloves, masks, and goggles when compelled to enter the sick room. Even today, some people still wonder whether they can catch the virus by using the computer keyboard of an infected fellow worker.

The most frightening misconception for many is the notion that being HIV-positive will rapidly lead to death. No matter how well-informed they are, many people believe the cliché, "HIV = AIDS = Death." They cannot conceive that years of health and productive work may lie ahead, that there will be good times, that much can still be learned. People who do not even have HIV-related symptoms may talk about quitting their jobs or selling their life insurance. The notion of future happiness is difficult to grasp, at least in the initial period after discovery of seropositive status.

Learning About HIV. Some people have lived in the midst of the epidemic for years, have cared for ill friends or lovers, and have been involved in community groups. They have seen their friends get sicker, and they know what the disease looks like. In contrast, a middle-class heterosexual woman who never met anyone with AIDS, and never imagined she might be personally involved, and even infected, has a lot to learn.

In some cases, people are familiar with the disease, but have never met or heard about HIV-positive people who are doing well. One woman, a former drug user who had been diagnosed in prison, said, "I had a brother who died of AIDS. I knew of women in prison who were dying. But I didn't have a positive role model. I didn't have anyone to say, 'Listen, I'm living with this. It's okay, you'll be okay.' I knew all the negative things that were happening, people getting really sick, people dying. People were scared, they were ashamed. All those things I knew. But I didn't have anything positive."

It isn't necessary to rush out and buy textbooks on HIV after being diagnosed as HIV-positive, but eventually it becomes important to educate oneself about symptoms and manifestations, what to worry about, and what to ignore. Even more important is knowing about trustworthy information sources, what kind of evidence to rely on and what to dismiss, and how to learn about new developments in diagnosis and treatment. There are national newsletters, local and national hotlines, a central government telephone number to find out about ongoing local experimental treatment trials, and computerized data bases offering free access to the scientific literature.

Identifying Community Resources. In most large and medium-sized cities, there are government-sponsored and volunteer social and support services available to those who are HIV-positive.

Community-based organizations and outreach programs offer seminars, workshops, and support groups to introduce people to the general topic of HIV illness. These services may include financial, nutritional, psychological, and spiritual advice and information. Large HIV epicenters offer a wide range of services. In Los Angeles, for example, there is a volunteer program called "Angel Food," and in New York City an equivalent program called "God's Love We Deliver." Both deliver hearty meals to the homebound on a day's notice, and do so without red tape for as long as needed. Some cities have programs to bring flowers to the sick, walk their dogs, provide escorts to medical appointments, and provide clergy for hospital visits or funeral services. Unfortunately, these services are not centrally coordinated and need to be contacted independently.

Government services, such as free medication programs or free transportation for the handicapped, may be available for people with AIDS. (Appendix I lists sources for payment assistance for many AIDS medications.) Again, to obtain needed services one has to learn what benefits are locally available, what is required in the way of eligibility and documentation, how to enroll, and how to maintain services once they are initiated. Food stamps, rent supplements, and monthly cash payments, as well as health services can be obtained by those people with AIDS who need such services and know how to get them, which often isn't easy. It helps to have friends who have already been there and can show the way. Ironically, people who have been on government assistance programs for many years are often more adept at negotiating government bureaucracies than are the middle-class or newly poor, who also eventually need such services.

No matter where people live, they can subscribe to both local and national newsletters about AIDS treatments and people with HIV illness. Such publications are of varying value and sophistication. Some are the best available sources about new studies, new findings, and novel treatments that seem promising, whereas others focus on what it is like to live with the virus. A new glossy magazine was launched in 1994 specifically for people with HIV illness: POZ: *The Magazine About Life and HIV*.

Adjustments in Lifestyle

Developing Healthy Habits. Some people discover their HIV-seropositive status as a consequence of changing their lifestyles, particularly if they have entered a drug or alcohol rehabilitation program where testing is encouraged. Others make the decision to reduce or eliminate excessive drug or alcohol use after they discover that they are HIV-positive. Although total abstinence is usually not necessary (unless one is so addicted that "a little bit" is never possible), moderating unhealthy habits and practices will certainly enhance health. When they discover they are HIV-positive, some people, initially despairing, go on alcohol or drug binges. However, most eventually decide to change their lives to protect their health. This includes eating regularly and sensibly, exercising, getting enough sleep, and using alcohol or other drugs only in moderation. It is at this point that people often try to eliminate or curb cigarette smoking, as well.

Planning for Change: Jobs, Insurance, Benefits. No major life decisions should be made immediately after discovering that one is HIV-positive. Rather than making radical changes all at once, it is better to merely think about and be prepared for change. This is especially true for people who have not yet been seriously ill.

Some people impulsively quit their jobs and spend their remaining time in recreational pursuits or hobbies. Much can be said for this attitude, but the problem of health insurance must be considered. Another drawback is that some people do not really have other pursuits and hobbies, and once having left work, become bored and listless. Instead of turning to freelance work or no work at all, it may be prudent at this time to consider seeking a job that includes health insurance and disability benefits. Financial decisions, such as management of resources, decisions about life insurance policies (i.e., obtaining partial cash reimbursement), transfer of property, and budgets, require careful attention. There are expert financial consultants who work on a voluntary or fee basis, and their advice may make a great difference in future financial security and access to medical resources.

FINDING SUPPORT

One of the most important messages people who discover they are HIV-positive need to hear is that *they are not alone*. A column with this title appears as the first article in every issue of a widely read monthly magazine called *Body Positive*, published in New York City. The article has been translated into five languages and reprinted in nearly 300 AIDS publications around the world. The central theme is, "You don't have to face this by yourself. There are lots of hands reaching out to assist you." The concluding passage is, "Just remember: those millions of people living successfully with HIV are people who've reached out to get the help they needed. Wherever you are, you can find support, or the means to create it. It just doesn't make sense for us to face the same issues without helping each other out. We are not alone. And neither are you."

Friends and Family

Family members are often, although not always, far more supportive and friendly than anticipated. Mothers and sisters are often more compassionate than brothers and fathers, although, of course, there are many exceptions. Some HIV-positive people complain, in fact, that they have to devote considerable energy to fending off solicitous efforts by their families, ranging from daily inquiries about their health, to urgent requests that they return to their (often distant) hometowns to be cared for by parents. Sometimes it helps to let parents visit and to answer their questions honestly. It can be reassuring for them to find that the person newly identified as HIV-positive is living his or her normal life in usual circumstances.

Some friends do drift away, which can happen with any illness or handicap. One man who became blind prior to developing AIDS said, "There was a mass exodus of friends from my life when I became blind. I didn't hear from anyone. It's just as well now, because if they couldn't handle blind, they certainly couldn't handle AIDS and blind." And some sexual partners cannot deal with the situation and depart. Friends may also behave inappropriately, providing paper plates and cups when the HIV-positive person visits, or asking them not to hug their children. Although more common in the early days of the epidemic, such behavior still occurs today, with more sophisticated rationalizations. Explaining why she wouldn't provide help and company to her HIV-positive gay brother who lived in the same city, far from any other relatives, an attorney said, "I can't help it, I have a germ phobia." For the most part, however, family and friends remain loyal, devoted, and committed.

Support Groups

Twelve-step programs, such as Alcoholics Anonymous, were among the first to identify and harness the power of support from others with similar problems. Self-help groups have become increasingly accepted for many different kinds of problems in our society, but perhaps nowhere more than in the AIDS community. In addition to providing direct services, such as therapeutic recreation, buddy programs, and educational materials, community-based agencies initiated the idea of support groups led by a "facilitator" (peer) rather than by an expert or professionally trained leader or therapist.

Most people with HIV illness sooner or later join a support group and often find great relief, encouragement, and motivation from their peers. One woman explained:

> There were a couple of things that happened when I was first diagnosed that really made me believe in God, that everything was going to be okay, that I wasn't totally forgotten by God. And one of the things was finding the support group. Right before I got thrush, I went to the movies with a friend and she invited a friend of a friend. I sat next to him, and we just started talking and getting along really great. And then I was diagnosed. My friend ran into him—he was HIV-positive—on the street the next day. And she told him, and he said, "I have this great place. Tell her to call me. And he really was totally there for me in the very beginning, and brought me to the support group, and got me hooked up with it. It made a big, big difference.

It isn't necessary for support group members to be exactly alike. The central issue in common is HIV illness. As a female attorney observed, "In the beginning, most women turned to GMHC or similar organizations [with predominantly gay clients] for advice, guidance, support. That's what I did initially, and I was very much involved with the gay community...I really made friends there. . . it's so different when there's somebody that's also going through it. There's just that certain level of being able to connect that you don't have with other people. But it's also very hard because you see the devastation. Somebody is always sick."

Once in a while, a particular group will be uncomfortable for someone. For example, a relatively asymptomatic HIV-positive man felt inhibited about describing his concerns because everyone else in the group was so much sicker, and his problems seemed comparatively trivial. Occasionally, gay men and drug users have trouble getting along in a group, but this is as often due to differences in needs and problems as to intolerance or dislike. Older men sometimes feel out of place and unwanted by the younger group members who predominate. They think the younger men have the attitude, "Well, you lived your life already. It's not a tragedy for you like it is for us." But of course, it is.

Support groups seem to be most helpful soon after discovery of HIV seropositivity. Group members can teach each other useful solutions to common problems, such as which pharmacies in town carry particular HIV medications at reasonable prices, how to keep track of multiple medications during the course of the day, where good meals are served in programs for people with AIDS, and what benefits are available from which agencies and how to obtain them. Many people feel guilty about burdening their healthy friends with their distress, and feel freer to express their misery and desperation about illness, current or prospective, to people who are also "in the trenches."

In large cities, one can sometimes find highly specialized support groups. For example, a special support group for HIV-positive visually impaired people exists within one New York City organization. There are support groups for partners or "care partners" of people with relatively advanced illness, for survivors of friends or family lost to AIDS. There are support groups for mothers of people with AIDS, for discharged prisoners with HIV illness, and for "sero-discordant couples" (where one is infected and the other is not).

Some support groups are designed to be short-term, often consisting of 12 weekly meetings. Members of such groups sometimes arrange to meet on their own after the group has formally ended. These are referred to as "closed" groups because only members attend. There are also "drop-in" groups, where the membership is constantly changing and there is no expectation of weekly attendance. Some closed groups go on for years, with all the advantages of a closely knit group that knows a great deal about what each has experienced, but with the drawback of having members get sick and die as time passes.

Adjusting Emotionally: The Role of the Professional Counselor

Most people manage to regain their psychological balance on their own, after the initial turmoil and distress associated with discovery of HIV-positive status. And, most people do not need psychiatric treatment just because they are HIV-positive. However, it may be very helpful to consult a counselor or therapist, if only briefly, particularly when there is no experience with HIV illness.

Therapists who work with HIV-positive people must be familiar with "the territory" and have an understanding of the course of HIV infection (see Chapter 12). For example, they should know what the prevalent issues are and how best to approach necessary tasks (including disclosure, education, and finding support groups and other community resources). As a rule, the focus of therapy is on current issues, rather than childhood memories, dream interpretation, or other material more suited to a leisurely psychoanalytic exploration of character and psychopathology. Credentials and professional training are important but cannot substitute for experience with other people who are HIV-positive. Acceptance of differing lifestyles is central.

REFERENCES

Hoover DR, Saah A, Bacellar H, et al. Clinical manifestations of AIDS in the era of pneumocystis prophylaxis. *New England Journal of Medicine.* 1993;329:1922-1926.

Leary WE. U.S. offers guide for doctors on care of those with HIV. *The New York Times.* 1994;January 21:A21.

Osmond D, Charlebois E, Lang W, et al. Changes in AIDS survival time in two San Francisco cohorts of homosexual men, 1983 to 1993. *Journal of the American Medical Association.* 1994;271:1083-1087.

Perry S, Jacobsberg L, Card C, et al. Severity of psychiatric symptoms after HIV testing. *American Journal of Psychiatry*. 1993;150:775-779.

Rabkin J, Remien R, Katoff L, et al. Suicidality in AIDS long term survivors: what is the evidence? *AIDS Care*. 1993; 5:401-411.

Weiss P, Wallace M, Olson P, et al. Changes in the mix of AIDS-defining conditions (letter). *New England Journal of Medicine*. 1993;329:1962.

8

BALANCING HOPE AND CANDOR IN LATE-STAGE ILLNESS

COMMENT
"Good" physicians give considerable thought to the processes and problems involved in communicating with patients about progressive illness and impending death. They are able to talk sensitively about issues in late-stage illness, such as the advisability of discontinuing procedures and/or medications. Although physicians differ in style, emphasis, and philosophy of treatment, most believe in being candid with patients as the end of life approaches. While he or she may not be able to offer hope of cure or even improvement, the good physician can help by providing both medical and emotional supportive care. Due to successful physician-patient communication, private patients with AIDS rarely spend their last days in a hospital intensive care unit.

New problems associated with managing late-stage illness have emerged during the last few years with the development of effective treatments for formerly fatal opportunistic infections. Mean survival after an AIDS diagnosis has been extended from about 12 weeks in 1981 or 1982 to 18 months or longer by the mid 1990s. By 1991, it was estimated that up to 15% of people with AIDS would live 3 or more years after diagnosis. A decade earlier, the likelihood of "long-term" survival was 5% to 10% (CDC data).

WHAT IS LATE-STAGE ILLNESS?

As people live longer, they may develop diseases that were previously uncommonly diagnosed (e.g., lymphoma and *Mycobacterium avium intracellulare* [MAI]). Hence, the task of medical management is becoming increasingly complex. During the months after diagnosis of an initial AIDS-defining condition, patients often return to their former level of health, especially after recovery from acute illnesses such as PCP (*Pneumocystis carinii* pneumonia) or toxoplasmosis. They may live for months or years feeling reasonably well, often working or actively engaging in volunteer activities. This period may or may not include discrete episodes of recurrent illness. There may or may not be gradual and progressive loss or deterioration of function. Eventually, however, a stage is reached where multiple systems may be involved, medications become less effective, and the overall picture shows clinical as well as silent disease progression in the absence of obvious remedies. This is the stage we define as "late." It is not determined by duration of survival after seroconversion or after an AIDS diagnosis, but by multiple and treatment-refractory symptomatology in conjunction with failing health.

A patient with late-stage illness, for example, may have loss of sight, taste, and smell from cytomegalovirus (CMV); neuropathy and accompanying loss of balance from HIV or CMV; nausea and vomiting of unidentified etiology; recurrent low-grade fevers; impaired bowel control; and some loss of verbal facility suggestive of mild cognitive impairment. Then acute pneumonia develops. Antibiotics may not be rapidly effective. Without additional aggressive treatment for the pneumonia, including mechanical ventilation, death appears imminent. The other problems would, however, remain even if the pneumonia remits.

A seemingly different scenario is that of the young person, with single digit CD4 cells, who has been plagued by a series of infections over a period of many months, although death does not appear imminent. Medications mount, as do medication side effects and dull, chronic pain, anorexia, and gastrointestinal distress that cannot be precisely diagnosed or treated. Analgesics relieve the pain but reduce alertness. Energy dwindles, and bed becomes the most comfortable place to be. Life becomes increasingly constricted, and despite the absence of an acute, immediately life-threatening illness, the days seem gray. There is no reason to anticipate improvement and every reason to expect further decline. This, too, is a late-stage patient who is not doing well.

Message, timing, and motive—what providers say and do, when, and why—become central issues when late-stage patients are not doing well. There is seldom a single, correct approach. The success of the health provider's communications often depends on style and context and a willingness to spend time explaining options. Moreover, the provider who makes an effort to become familiar with patients' beliefs, social ties, and financial resources can be especially effective and comforting. Balancing personal style with that of the patient is part of the practitioner's art. While there is always a need to take into account specific circumstances, patient characteristics, and other unique factors, it is useful to study general philosophies of "successful" patients and physicians. The absence, or failure, of delicate communications at this point can constitute a major source of anger and distress for patients and those close to them. In this chapter, we focus on what physicians actually say to their patients, in the event that standard treatments have not been effective or do not exist. We also address what "good" physicians say to patients, and their loved ones, as death approaches.

MAINTAINING HOPE

Hope is an essential element of living with prolonged, severe illness. Hope has two components: a positive focus and a future orientation. Jerome Frank (1973), a pioneer among psychiatrists in identifying the therapeutic roles of hope and persuasion in healing, defined hope "as the perceived possibility of achieving a goal." In health and in youth, we tend to look at distant temporal horizons. With advancing age or illness, the future frame shortens. Even in extreme circumstances, hope may shrink but it need not disappear altogether. One can think positively ahead to the coming week, the coming day, or even the coming hour.

Almost all physicians believe that it is possible to maintain hope while being truthful with patients, even when their prospects are poor. The first requirement, however, is that the physician maintains hope. That hope can then be communicated to the patient. This is largely achieved by shifting goals and focusing on helping patients achieve their own (realistic) wishes in the time left to them. This usually entails a shift of objective from cure to providing comfort and eventually to addressing the process of dying rather than its timing. One physician described the process this way:

> I can maintain hope in my own mind, but what I hope for changes. The challenge, for me, is to get a fix on my concept of what reality is or will be for this person and change their perception of reality to match mine. I try to redirect their hope. When people come to realize that they are going to die, what they are most concerned about is what that is going to be like. That is where you can instill some hope because you can make it clear you are not going to abandon them when the time comes. You can deal with concrete issues: "It won't be painful;" "It won't be frightening;" and "We won't leave you." I think there can be hope in that, too.

Another physician put it simply: "If there's nothing I can change about what's happening to them, there is something I can change about how they relate to it."

Difficult clinical decisions can be tempered with positive examples and anecdotes to help patients maintain hope.

One physician explained that, even in late-stage (but not acute) illness:

> I never take away the hope that a new advance may come. The odds of that happening in the next 2 to 4 years for HIV are low, but it could happen. MAI is a case in point. Until recently, MAI was deliberately not treated simply because, 'What was the point? Nothing worked.' Now, a whole new range of drugs such as clarithromycin, azithromycin, and ansamycin [now called rifabutin], have come along to change that. By the same token, I warn patients not to count on a cure.

This physician emphasized that one should let the patient "lead" in terms of the amount of information they want to hear. Others also indicated that explicit questions should be answered directly, but that additional information need not necessarily be volunteered.

THE HAZARDS OF OPTIMISM

Although physicians generally seek to instill and maintain optimism in their patients, they also consider themselves responsible for realistically delivering accurate information. At times, these missions become incompatible. In early illness, it is appropriate to emphasize optimism. For patients who are not doing well, however, the conflict between hope and candor can be more difficult. Intentional overstatement of the positive can have significant costs, e.g., patients may delay making necessary plans or may lose confidence in the physician. On the other hand, diminution of the patient's hope can significantly diminish determination to keep going, as well as reduce the quality of remaining life.

Physicians are keenly aware of this dilemma. As one doctor said, "There have been occasions when I am overly optimistic because of personal involvement and an inability to be truly frank. It becomes difficult and is one of the dangers of treating friends or becoming friends with patients." Another physician observed, "I never offer hope where I think hope is totally not based in reality, but I always try to operate from the assumption that if there is anything objective that is positive, even if it is an extreme exception, I want the person to know." Finally, another physician said, "I think I am always very realistic. The further we get along to the terminal event, the more accurate I am, but I always throw in that I believe in miracles."

Believing in miracles or "magic," can be problematic in that there is a fine line between magic and denial. Sometimes there is no line at all. A minister who works with people with AIDS admitted, "I don't believe in miracles. I don't let myself. To fall in with the patient's denial is comforting at the time, but then when the rug comes out, it comes out from under both of us. If I'm scrambling to regain my equilibrium when they are trying to get theirs, it makes me a little useless."

Another pitfall of undue optimism was voiced by a physician who said, "I am aware of the temptation to be overly positive. I try not to mislead patients out of cowardice or kindness, but the majority of people are in a very gray and murky area. I don't think in this disease that accuracy is frequently legitimate or appropriate. You can't be that accurate."

NO MORE PROCEDURES

A 1992 editorial published by the *New England Journal of Medicine* discussed the options facing patients and physicians who are involved with medically grave situations for which available treatments have not worked (Campion, 1992):

> For any disease, there is a limited number of treatments that are known to be effective. When those fail, the physician has to consider alternatives that are either new and unproved or ancient and of uncertain benefit. After enduring a chronic disease and failing to respond to the standard therapies,

patients can become desperate...research helps protect desperate patients from useless procedures. But there will always be urgent situations in which it is tempting to try them anyway. Then decisions must be empirical but not arbitrary. And it is probably true that sometimes, if rarely, "Diseases desperate grown, by desperate appliance are relieved" (Shakespeare, Hamlet, Act IV, scene 3).

For a number of late-stage, AIDS-related conditions, not even the first of these assumptions is true—there are no established, consistently effective treatments. Success in forestalling or treating opportunistic infections, such as cryptococcal meningitis or PCP, may lead to the subsequent emergence of an infection less amenable to treatment, such as cryptosporidiosis or progressive wasting of unknown origin. When interventions fail, the problem becomes how far to pursue other medical interventions and when or whether a decision should be made to discontinue aggressive medical treatments altogether. If such a decision is reached or is under consideration, the question then arises as to whether and when it is appropriate to say so to the patient.

It may be useful to begin by asking the patient how things are going. Patients often understand their situation and may indicate that they realize that nothing has worked, that the quality of life is not acceptable, and that they are ready to stop. It is better for the patient to arrive independently at this understanding than to hear it from someone else.

Sometimes the physician has to clarify where the patient is, what has been attempted, what the outcomes have been thus far, and what the remaining options are. A physician might say, "We did this, we did that, and things don't seem to be better. What do you think?" The physician could then add, "We are at a stage in your illness where you will have greater problems. The medicines will be less effective. Sometimes at this stage, people decide to make things simpler and gear their treatment toward comfort, rather than trying to fix the underlying problem or trying to live as long as possible." It should be very clear that the discussion is about shifting the type of care rather than terminating care. One physician pointed out that, "I also explicitly say something about pain control, which is often a big fear. Sometimes people will bring up the subject of assisted suicide. I think it's important to let the person talk about that, whether you believe in it or not, because sometimes they just need to know that if things go badly, you'll do your best to keep them comfortable."

Some physicians are explicit:

> Our tendency is to be honest, sometimes brutally honest. Generally we'll work someone up and keep doing tests and trying different interventions until we can't think of anything else to try. Then we always sit down with the patient and say: "This is a hard conversation for me to have with you. You are not doing well. You need to know what is going through our minds. We've done this test and that test, and we've poked and prodded

you, and we can't think of anything else to do that will make a difference. We want to continue to make you as comfortable as possible, but we don't think there's anything more we can do that's going to make a very big difference."

While this message is honorable in intent, we disagree with the central message, namely that "there's nothing more we can do that's going to make a very big difference." Prolonging survival is not the only big difference that a physician can offer. Dying without loss of dignity or control, where and with whom one wishes, can also make a very big difference. In that context, there may not be additional technical procedures to perform, but there is a great deal that the physician can still do to help the patient achieve a comfortable and peaceful death.

At the other extreme, some physicians resist the assumption that a decision should ever be made to discontinue medical treatments altogether. "There is always something experimental," one such physician claimed, "something you haven't tried. I ask the patient, 'Is it worth it to you to try anything else?' Because if they want me to keep working, I'll keep working, if there's any quality of life at all. I think most people are pretty real as they approach the end. They just don't want to suffer any more." A self-described cockeyed optimist said, "I think everything is treatable. I'm always looking for an answer. So, I don't say, 'You're going blind from CMV.' I say, 'You've got CMV. Now we've got to make you better.'" This physician was willing to acknowledge, however, that a colleague had been too aggressive in treating a dying patient who had no real hope.

One physician explained that his decision to discontinue medical tests and treatments was contingent on his understanding of the patient's condition:

> If someone has been declining and wasting, has MAI and CMV and all the advanced HIV diseases, and they're dying, I let them know that [and I stop aggressive treatment]. It is a much easier decision because it is part of the predictable course of the illness. But if the person is doing poorly and I am at my wit's end because the person has an undiagnosed illness and is deteriorating, I try to find out what is going on as aggressively as I can and perhaps get a second opinion.

Some physicians say they are still unsure about the best course to take in such instances:

> I always believed in intubating my patients. I always believed in being very aggressive. With early-stage disease, there is no question in my mind. But now what happens with end-stage disease? What happens when you know someone has got KS [Kaposi's sarcoma] in the lungs, your chemotherapy is not working, and he doesn't want to give up? Do you intubate? I have done that. My rationalization was that if someone was that sick and you intubated him, he would be on the tube 24 or 48 hours before dying. You're

not incurring any massive, chronic care expenses as you would if you keep a stroke victim alive for months and months on a respirator. But, I am beginning to rethink my aggressive stance. Is that the way a person should die—on a respirator, maybe tied down? The hard part for me is when the patient asks you to do everything, even when I know it is not going to work.

The timing and certainty of the decision to forgo further new active treatments is not always apparent. "It is sometimes hard to know when you've reached the end of the line," one physician pointed out. "And usually when you have, the patient is so sick, he doesn't need to be told." In contrast, another doctor said, "I think I'm pretty confident about when the point of no return has been reached. Once that point has been reached, I usually am very forthright. I may not speak with the patient because he may not be competent at that point, but I'll be straightforward about the situation. I'll speak to the loved one or responsible party and just lay it all out. At that point, I stop aggressive treatment." Nevertheless, even this doctor would not actually say, "There is nothing more we can do," nor would it be true. Instead, as many others have indicated, he switches gears, and when he feels he has no further medical options and perceives that the patient is dying, he is likely to make a home visit. At that point, he is offering comfort and support instead of further diagnostic and treatment procedures.

Nearly all physicians acknowledge that in many instances a point is reached when additional diagnostic procedures or more medications are not likely to be useful. They strongly believe, however, that they can still make significant contributions to patient care by providing physical and emotional comfort. Further, there is virtual consensus that patients know what is happening: "They've seen so many die. They usually figure things out for themselves."

No More Medicine

At some point, when the patient is no longer responding to multiple medications, the question of whether and/or when to discontinue medication will arise. Since HIV medications often have significant side effects, it may seem, in the absence of therapeutic effects, that the patient could be more comfortable without them. For patients with multi-system disease, who may be taking as many as 40 pills daily plus infusions, a time comes when the quality of life may be (transiently) enhanced with less, rather than more, treatment. Nevertheless, although the difference between not initiating additional procedures or medications and discontinuing current medications may seem subtle, the implications can be perceived quite differently.

First, physicians do not always tell the patients about procedures they have decided not to initiate; whereas, patients are perfectly aware of ongoing treatments that may be stopped. Second, whether or not to initiate a new treatment may be considered by the patient a matter of strategy; whereas, the suggestion to stop ongoing medications may be taken as a message that the situation is hopeless. The underlying issue is whether the recommendation to discontinue medication is inherently demoralizing or worth trying, with the goal of reducing physically uncomfortable side effects.

Most physicians view discontinuation of medication as prudent and offer this option to patients. As one doctor explained:

> With advancing illness you get less benefit with each increment or new drug. It's very, very clear that at some point, the risks and discomforts and disadvantages of giving people 15 medicines outweigh any benefits. I am very comfortable holding back on anything that isn't really essential. If someone has seizures, I leave them on seizure medications. Or, if they have pain, I treat it. But three-quarters of the drugs they are on are dispensable.

Similarly, another physician said:

> As long as there is some reasonable expectation of recovery or amelioration you can try to get patients to tolerate side effects. But I actually have begun to negotiate with some patients about whether or not they would like to be withdrawn from all medications, other than I.V. fluids and oxygen. When death is imminent, the odds of an antibiotic, for example, doing any good are pretty low. By stopping the drug, you just might reduce side effects and enhance quality of life. Someone with a week to live won't die more quickly because you take him off his TB medication. It doesn't work that way. I suggest simplifying the treatment regimen when death is imminent.

There are some physicians who decline to make such a recommendation because of its psychological impact. One explained, "That has the feeling of giving up to me." He acknowledged that he sometimes discontinues nutritional supplements (TPN): "That is as close as I'll come to letting the patient know they've reached a point where the fight is over."

Some patients do react quite poorly when advised to stop taking their medications. In one instance, a patient was obviously dying but didn't choose to deal with it or discuss the subject with his doctor, who didn't bring it up either. He complained constantly about all the side effects of the drugs he was taking. His physician finally told him, "You know, you can stop taking all of them. They're not doing any good." A friend of the patient recalled: "I'll never forget that day. That's when J. decided to die. He said his doctor had just told him he was dying. That was one of the saddest times for him psychologically. He was not ready for that news."

The problem here seems to have been that the patient's message was not heard. Perhaps he wasn't asking to stop the medications but needed validation that the side effects were really unpleasant. Another possible response might have been, "Yes, the side effects are terrible. Why do you continue to do this?" Overall, despite the risk of demoralization, most physicians advise patients to discontinue medications when they seem ineffective.

So Little Time

Although most physicians refuse to predict the amount of time a patient may have left, the general consensus is that he or she should be told when death is imminent. Practical reasons for this include the need for patients to take care of their affairs promptly (e.g., appoint health proxies, write wills, sign "do not resuscitate" [DNR] orders) if they have not already done so and to indicate whether they would prefer to die at home or in hospital and who they want to have with them at the end.

One physician offered this script: "We say, 'You are doing very poorly. We don't think you're going to make it through this, and we need to know where you want to be. You know if you go home and you want to come back, that's fine. We need to know if you've made a decision about where you want to die and who you want to be with.' " Another physician was less blunt. "I might say, 'I will be honest with you that we're not being successful.' I don't tell them that they are about to die."

A somewhat different approach was offered by a physician who said:

> Sometimes I have to explain to people that they are much further advanced in their HIV disease than they were 6 months ago, that things are different, that I'm not sure that lots of tests and lots of procedures are indicated, and that I would just try to make them as comfortable as I can. When I put it that way, they get the message and usually agree. Very few patients disagree and insist on being aggressive. There are only so many times you can do a biopsy or a colonoscopy. Enough is enough.

Another physician explained:

> A particular situation that comes to mind is when a patient has progressive respiratory distress, is heading toward respiratory arrest, and hasn't addressed the issue of DNR. I'll say, "Look, this is a situation where you have to make up your mind." I'll tell them that I strongly recommend they sign a DNR order: "I don't think there's much hope of ever coming off a respirator once you get on it. And, I think if you get on a respirator, you're going to be very uncomfortable and heavily sedated until you die. By postponing death, we are not keeping you alive." So I am honest.

A complication of late-stage illness that may render these issues particularly difficult is cognitive impairment. One physician observed that "in these extreme situations patients are infrequently crystal clear in their thinking." Another specifically mentioned dementia as an increasingly common characteristic of late-stage illness. In such cases, it is important that the physician go over the issues with the family, partner, or lover.

Despite a widely shared belief in the appropriateness of candor, virtually all physicians caution against making absolute statements. As one put it, "Even if the outlook is poor, we should always maintain a glimmer of hope. People do surprise us. I think one can be honest and forthright without being totally pessimistic."

PHYSICAL COMFORT, SYMPTOM CONTROL, AND EMOTIONAL SUPPORT

When the physician does not believe further treatments would be useful, attention is usefully directed at supportive care—nutrition, pain relief, toileting, comfort. This can be time consuming, difficult, and frustrating, especially if the patient wishes to be home. Nevertheless, one physician believes that "the major aim of the physician should be to try to keep the person at home . . . it's actually a lot of work to coordinate all the nursing support and the social work, etc., that constitute good care." Another physician spoke of the frustrations of trying to make such arrangements with home care agencies, of obtaining authorization from insurance companies, and of making sure that all the necessary components of supportive care (e.g., pharmaceutical supplies, home attendants, visiting nurses) are in place. While these tasks are not taught in medical school, nor are they part of the physician's role historically, they are clearly essential to patients' wellbeing. Some AIDS specialists handle this problem by employing additional office staff who take on such responsibilities.

Under the best of circumstances, arrangements for home nursing care, for pharmaceutical supplies, and a home attendant are managed by the physician's office. Often, however, these tasks are left to friends and family. A guide for arranging home care is provided in Appendix II.

PAIN RELIEF

Since fear of pain is common as death approaches, the issue of pain relief looms large. "I always try to offer at least one guarantee, which is 'We will not let you suffer.' I'm proud that I have become nothing less than a master of using neuroleptics, narcotics, sedatives, and tranquilizers, and I cannot tell you how enthusiastic I am that we learn more."

Many physicians have become quite adept at explaining to the patient (and family) their understanding that the time has come to desist from aggressive treatments and to focus on comfort, which often includes pain management. At this point, however, when the patient is at home, often with care that the doctor helped to organize, his or her role may become ambiguous. Arrangements are made through the home health agency. Some physicians make a deliberate effort to maintain direct contact with the patient, although most do not. One physician makes a point of using the telephone to stay in touch: "You don't have to phone every day, but the occasional call helps, especially when things are not going very well. If people lose interest, the patient feels everyone is just waiting for him or her to die, and I think that [perception] is a real killer." Another physician actually carries with him a "worry list" of eight or ten patients he is currently concerned about, and calls them regularly.

While such behavior seems reasonable and appropriate, it is uncommon. The pressure of work, the lack of time, the competing demands of acutely sick patients often mean that the HIV specialist may not be able to return patient phone calls until 8 or 9 P.M., much less initiate calls to patients they haven't heard from. Then, too, not every HIV specialist conceptualizes this as something they should be doing. Finally, the reward is low and there are costs, not only in terms of time but also in having to confront patients one cannot cure despite professional training and experience. It is the exceptional physician who pauses to follow through in this manner.

TIME AT THE BEDSIDE

Hospitalized patients and their families sometimes worry that once aggressive treatment is discontinued, the physician will lose interest in their case. And sometimes that is true. The physician may no longer feel it necessary to visit, to stop by, to talk. This may be due to the physician's understanding of his or her role, or to a reluctance to visit a "treatment failure."

During active phases of treatment, there are diagnostic procedures for the physician to interpret, tests to order, treatments to establish. When the doctor is seeking cure, or at least amelioration or remission, visiting the patient and engaging in conversation is often less informative for diagnostic purposes than looking at laboratory results and films. However, when there are no additional technical interventions, the bedside visit assumes central importance and meaning to patient, family, and friends. Lewis Thomas (1992, p 48) pointed out that this historically has been what physicians did:

> The doctor's real role during all those centuries, was more like that of a professional friend, someone at the bedside, standing by. When he was called a therapist, it was more in the etymological sense of the original Greek therapon... In its ancient meaning, it carries all the obligations that medicine and the other health professions have for patients with AIDS: to stand by, to do whatever can be done, to comfort, and to run all the risks that doctors have always run in times of plague.

TALKING TO FRIENDS AND FAMILY

Most very sick patients have at least one caring person at their bedside, and sometimes the hospital room is crowded. "Their social network is something to envy," said one physician who was too overworked to have a social life of his own. "A guy goes in the hospital, and I go to make rounds, and there are eight people there at every moment of the day. A guy will give up his job to go take care of this other one who is sick, and this one is a care partner for that one, it is unbelievable." Although the ranks of dedicated friends may thin with the mounting toll of the epidemic and the cumulative weariness of survivors, still, there are usually caring people at the bedside when the end is near.

These people cannot be ignored, for their own sakes as well as that of the patient. Sometimes incongruous combinations of people surround the patient: urban lover and gay friends may be meeting biological family members from rural America for the first time. Sometimes these relatives had never visited the city before, nor been in close touch with their "wayward" child or sibling. It is usually family members who come to the city; when very sick people go home to small towns to be taken care of by their families, their former friends are seldom called to be present at the end. The family may not know who they are, how to contact them, or may not care to involve them.

Under the best of circumstances, the physician has met at least one of these people earlier in the course of the patient's care. Lovers or spouses often accompany each other on outpatient visits, and sometimes friends or family (most often a mother or sister) ask or are invited to come along. If at these earlier occasions the patient doesn't take responsibility for bringing them into the consultation, an alert physician will notice them in the waiting room and invite them in, even if briefly. It relieves the anxiety of these others to meet the physician who is caring for their loved one, to develop confidence in him or her, and even to feel comfortable calling the doctor directly (with the patient's consent) for explanation or reassurance.

When the patient becomes very ill, these "significant others" also need to know what is happening, what is expected, and how they can be helpful. If the patient becomes unable to participate in his or her own care, friends and family may be called on to articulate and/or carry out their wishes. However, when families seem overwhelmed, the physician may need to help them take time off to forestall their exhaustion or burnout. As Klagsbrun (1982) observed in his comments to nonpsychiatric practitioners, "You may have to 'order' the family members to limit their help and their visits [or bedside vigil if the patient is at home] in order to prevent them from abusing themselves... Their feelings of guilt may not permit them to limit their time at the bedside unless you take responsibility for doing so." Klagsbrun also speaks of the importance of the physician spending time with patient and family "without feeling called upon to be falsely encouraging. Your presence is what counts, not your false promises or empty encouragement."

When the patient is very sick, the physician may actually turn to those around him for some sense of the patient's, and their, wishes. One said as much: "I usually try to get a feel for how the patient would like me to proceed. I also listen to family, to friends. It almost becomes a consensus decision. If everyone is totally exhausted and the patient really just wants to be let alone and die, I go along with that if I think I can't bring the patient back. If everyone is willing to fight, I fight."

Sometimes even medical decisions take loved ones into account. In discussing pain management at the end of life, one physician noted:

> You must not use analgesics and sedatives in such a way as to deny the family the opportunity for closure with hugs and kisses and conversations and hand squeezing or whatever is part of the dying process. To have the family sit wringing their hands while the patient is in a deep coma induced by a doctor I don't think is fair. There should be a balance. And the beauty about drugs like morphine is that we know how to use them to achieve that balance.

NEGOTIATING THE DYING PROCESS

At some point, it is likely that the physician and patient will acknowledge that "enough is enough." Sometimes this means discontinuation of medical procedures and drugs. In other cases, I.V. morphine may be started with the double purpose of alleviating pain and, possibly, accelerating the timing of impending death. After its initiation, there may be a period of alertness for several days, or even weeks, before death occurs.

During this period, it may be helpful to ask loved ones or family members, "Is there something you haven't said? Are there things you need to say? Have you said that maybe it is okay to go now?" And it may be necessary to tell the lover or relatives, "Let him know you'll be okay, that you'll be taken care of and things are fine." A newspaper obituary illustrates this clearly:

> Ms. G's health had deteriorated since spring. During the final days, her three closest friends, parents, and grandmother gathered by her bedside. "We were encouraging her not to fight, because she was such a fighter, and not to struggle, to let go," said one of her friends. Finally, when her three friends began laughing over old stories at her bedside in an abrupt departure from the grim mood that had prevailed there, Ms. G. began to slip away. "I think she knew that we were going to be all right, and decided it was OK to go," said her friend (Obituary, 1992).

Finally, it may be necessary to assist the family in making plans so that they can start the process of letting go. "Did you make the funeral arrangements yet?" The professional can and should raise certain issues that will engage family and friends in the process of transition.

In summary, despite differences in style, emphasis, and philosophy, most physicians prefer to be candid about illness status, to speak of the possibility of impending death, and arrangements to be made. At the same time, these professionals never cease giving reassurance about supportive care, both practical and emotional.

REFERENCES

Campion EW. Desperate diseases and plasmapheresis (editorial). *New England Journal of Medicine*. 1992;326:1425-1427.

Frank J. *Persuasion and Healing: A Comparative Study of Psychotherapy*, rev ed, Baltimore: Johns Hopkins University Press; 1973.

Klagsbrun S. The management of the dying patient and death. In: Kornfeld D, Finkel J, (eds) *Psychiatric Management for Medical Practitioners*. New York: Grune and Stratton; 1982, pp 447-460.

Obituary. *The New York Times*. 1992; October 8: p D24.

Thomas L. *The Fragile Species*. New York: Scribner; 1992, p 48.

9

WHEN PHYSICIANS CAN'T CURE PATIENTS

COMMENT

The intellectual and emotional incentives of HIV medicine appear to be substantial and are widely shared by practitioners. Nevertheless, physicians who treat HIV-positive patients are vulnerable to both work overload and emotional stress. Restructuring certain logistic aspects of a practice may relieve at least some of these stressors and prevent "burnout."

Physicians who can maintain a sense of control over their professional lives; who have a wide perspective on a patient's overall course; who can anticipate death and manage dying well; who have developed appropriate personal escape mechanisms; and who have settled on the degree of closeness to their patients that makes them comfortable are most likely to continue to work effectively as AIDS specialists.

Those outside the field often wonder how AIDS specialists manage to keep going despite seeing the decline and often the deaths of large numbers of very ill patients. In medical school, students are taught to cure patients, or at least to effect long-term amelioration of their symptoms. Only a small part of the curriculum is devoted to management of patients with progressive, fatal disease. Nevertheless, the incentives and rewards of an HIV practice exist, although they are not nearly as obvious to observers as are the stressors.

REWARDS—THE "HIGHS"

Clinical Success

HIV specialists are extremely articulate and enthusiastic about the incentives intrinsic to their work. Surprisingly, the most frequently cited reward is clinical success. One physician explained, "I make people better sometimes. And I keep them better, until nature makes it impossible for me to keep them better." He went on to observe that "...this is probably the last place where medicine is still an art. You have to use every last ounce of skill and sense. It's challenging because there is no textbook." Another physician pointed out that many battles are won during the course of the disease and that there is only one defeat. Yet another emphasized that treating AIDS patients is "...the most demanding and interesting work a physician can do. You have to know a lot of medicine to take care of AIDS patients, and you have to keep up with it."

New Developments

Another exciting aspect of AIDS medicine is the speed with which new insights and treatments are being developed. "Treating patients with AIDS really involves cutting edge medicine. Medical technologies that were just concepts ten years ago are already in use today." The sense of real progress being made against a terrible foe is powerful. As one physician noted, "We have made vast strides in this disease with drugs developed as a specific response to the AIDS epidemic. That's a huge source of satisfaction."

Physician/Patient Relationship

Having the opportunity to interact with this group of patients is experienced —and expressed—by many physicians as deeply satisfying: "I can't imagine how brave they are. The vast majority are incredible inspirations;" "A larger source of satisfaction comes from the spiritual side, namely to see patients fight this disease with the strength of their inner resources...;" "The main satisfaction is taking care of people who are very much interested in taking care of themselves...."

In addition, most HIV specialists develop special relationships with their patients. One explained, "It's one of the few instances in medical care where you can have a long-term close relationship with your patients, making a major difference in the quality of their lives and care." An HIV clinic director noted, "AIDS doctors say that they like the relationships they build with patients and often the gratitude, the sense that they're doing something for somebody whom other people would not even consider taking care of."

Overall Satisfaction

The "highs," or satisfactions, of treating AIDS patients certainly include the many clinical successes, participation in the "cutting edge" of medicine, the exploration of a variety of medical areas, and the development of warm and rewarding relationships with patients. Most physicians, though, may experience an unexpected personal growth in addition to these other rewards. One physician offered a particularly vivid description of the rewards of HIV medicine:

> I've learned a lot of technical things. I've become a smarter doctor. This work has reinforced for me the great good a primary care doctor can do. I've gotten to meet specialists I wouldn't have met because of the vast range of problems my patients have had. I've gotten to do a lot of teaching. I've developed a sense of expertise in a particular area. I get to do something that means a lot to me in terms of my community. And it makes me think about big issues. It's easy not to think about ethical or spiritual

things when someone has a simple urinary tract infection, but you're really facing it when your patient has become fecally incontinent. On a medical level, that's not a big deal compared to pneumonia, but psychologically, for that person, it's an incredibly big deal. And AIDS has taught me the difference between dealing with pathophysiology and with the person the pathophysiology is in.

In my own life, it has made me place more value on living day to day, and it has made me appreciate simple things more. I can look at a piece of art now and get tears in my eyes. It has given me a sense that I'm doing something that matters. It has made me healthier in terms of taking care of myself, because I recognize how incredibly stressed out I can get. So, it has almost been like an Outward Bound trip for a doctor.

STRESSORS—THE "LOWS"

Although similar to other medical specialties, the practice of HIV medicine may be particularly stressful in a number of specific ways, including the sheer volume of work, bureaucratic regulations and paperwork, and economic and time costs. Here, we review some of the strategies doctors use to maintain their enthusiasm, morale, and commitment to HIV medicine.

Too Much to Do, Too Little Time

Perhaps the most pervasive complaint among HIV specialists concerns the sheer volume of work—a sense of unremitting pressure, of urgency without relief. One physician we met, who had become so overwhelmed by work pressure and personal conflicts that he actually left practice for a while, now has a reduced schedule and reports no pressure of work. Most others cite this as a major problem in their daily lives. The corollary of this perceived pressure is a sense of being out of control.

Physical exhaustion seems to be a universal experience at some point in every practice. Some of the more senior physicians have learned to live with this problem by deliberately reorganizing their lives and practices. Others, however, describe their lives as consumed by their work. Feeling overburdened and lacking support staff and/or weekend coverage has led some physicians to seriously contemplate changing fields.

One physician explained that people quit this work because of patient overload: "You cannot predict the amount of work you're going to have with a patient, the number of hours you really need to devote. And the illness is something that is going to require hospitalization. So if you think you can be locked in an office, that's probably not going to work. And, you need a group of co-workers [to share coverage]."

Another specialist referred to the cumulative emotional and physical demands and said, "Basically, I just can't take it any more. It's just too much. I've been doing it for years. I'm tortured. I don't sleep. I haven't slept in 5 years. I can't keep up the lifestyle any more. I just don't have the strength. Physically, I can't do it."

The line between physical and emotional fatigue clearly gets blurred, but the sheer volume of work that some of these physicians undertake appears extraordinary. Some feel guilty about taking time off, even to attend to routine chores. "This guy is dying, and I'm getting a haircut." On the other hand, some physicians have learned to moderate their schedules. Others have turned to research or other activities that are less insatiable.

Even when physicians take major steps to reduce the pressure of their work by restructuring the way they carry out their practices (e.g., refusing new patients, hiring an associate physician or physician assistant, arranging for others to be the primary admitting physician for hospitalizations), there is the reality that the volume of work, the unanticipated exigencies, and the urgency of care combine to produce high levels of pressure.

Regulation and Bureaucracy

The other major stressor that plagues all health care professionals is increasing governmental and bureaucratic regulation. This seems particularly salient in AIDS medicine, however, because of the high cost and unproven nature of many AIDS treatments. According to one physician, "What is going to happen and what has already happened in terms of the loss of control in health care delivery is mind-boggling. Just in the last 2 months, the way health care is being fashioned and controlled by insurance companies and government is coming down very negatively on the physician."

Time, Money, and Medical Costs

The practice of AIDS medicine may be particularly affected by increasing regulatory interference for a number of reasons. First, people with HIV illness often require longer office visits, because they present with more complicated medical conditions, because treatment options are less clear-cut and require more extensive discussions between doctor and patient, and because people who are very sick often need more attention from their physicians. AIDS physicians are likely to get involved with their patients and to have closer relationships than are most other practitioners. Moreover, the patient's spouse or "significant other" may play a part in the patient's health care support, which also takes time. Longer patient visits are not generally reimbursed appropriately and are not "cost effective" for the physician.

A second consideration, not unique to AIDS medicine but particularly pertinent, is the need to obtain experimental medications. The use of non-marketed medications often requires considerable paperwork at the very least, and in some cases, enrollment of patients in clinical trials of experimental medications. This process often obligates the physician to obtain approval from his or her local institution's human subjects review committee.

A third aspect of AIDS medicine that is costly is the need for the physician to also function as a social worker, including handling the extensive paperwork involved in applying for and maintaining benefits. And the treating physician in private practice is at least partially responsible for dealing with the insurance companies, municipal services, and home care programs his or her patients interact with.

While insurers and government program officers are increasing surveillance of medical costs in all specialties, AIDS medicine is particularly vulnerable because many treatments are spectacularly expensive. One form of home infusion for CMV (cytomegalovirus) retinitis and other CMV conditions can be billed at more than $12,000 a month, not including nursing services, and the treatment is usually required for life. Other medications are also notoriously expensive.

Insurance companies recently have begun to refuse to pay for more costly medicines when less expensive (adequate but less effective or with more side effects) medicines may be substituted. As one physician noted, HMOs and insurance carriers are not accustomed to large bills for laboratory tests and treatments on an ongoing basis because they have little experience with very sick people who need long-term, often lifelong management. Overall, the practice of AIDS medicine is likely to be increasingly regulated on the basis of financial considerations.

HOW PHYSICIANS MANAGE STRESS

Experienced AIDS physicians use several strategies to prevent emotional exhaustion and deal with patient deaths. These include both psychological techniques and practical methods for arranging their professional practices and their personal lives (see, "Practical Tips for Physicians," page 115).

Anticipatory Mourning

Among the psychological strategies often cited by physicians, the most common is anticipatory mourning. One doctor explained, "I've developed a protective mechanism that allows me to remain in control, so that I'm not surprised...over the years I think of a lot of patients that I have as already dead. There comes a point, which is different for individual patients, where they cross a line. That's when I know I've lost them. When that happens, I start grieving. By the time death actually occurs, I'm okay. I find this very helpful so that when people get very sick at the end of their illness, I'm prepared for it." In this way, grieving is more diffuse and takes place over a period of time in preparation for the eventual death.

This appears to be a widespread phenomenon. At a certain point, when the caregiver arrives at the perception that the patient is going to die in the foreseeable future, an internal shift takes place. One doctor described it as "removing my intimacy to a certain degree. Hopefully not in a way that the patient will perceive."

The crucial skill here is to be able to engage in this process of anticipatory mourning—which evidently is effective for the physician—without communicating to the patient a change in attitude that leads to a feeling of abandonment. Without this delicate balance, a strategy that works for the physician may generate further distress in patients already on a downwardly spiraling course of illness.

Reframing or Shifting Gears

"Reframing" means changing the way you look at a phenomenon. It is a technique taught by psychologists trained in cognitive therapy. Recognizing that providing good medical care can be as much about enhancing quality of life as about prolonging life is an important way of reframing one's role when treating patients with a progressive and life-threatening disease.

Reframing can be done from the outset, when a person is first seen by the physician. Instead of seeing him or herself as responsible for "making the patient better," which is the usual objective in medicine, the physician's role can be redefined. "I look at things as a process. I hope for every HIV-positive patient I work with that he or she may be one of the lucky ones who does well. But I also accept from the outset that they may pass away within 6 months, 2 years, or 5 years. I try to frame my care as helping and being with them on their journey wherever that takes them. The only way I can make sense of this tragedy is to give people the best care possible."

In this context, death is seen as part of the journey, instead of a failure. Managing death well for the patient and the family can become a positive goal. When it is done well, it, too, can be a gratifying experience. "When you know you are powerless to change things, at least make it easier for people, make their deaths easier."

One physician told of a patient who had a prolonged hospitalization with a number of end-stage illnesses. "It became apparent after an aggressive trial of therapy that he was not going to get better. He made it very clear that he wanted to go home and die. So we arranged for him to go home and die in a comfortable, warm, clean, pain-free environment. I felt really good about that…even though the patient died, we won that battle."

Adjusting goals in this manner is predicated on acknowledgement that there is a time for someone to die. Not all physicians, consultants, or patients endorse this view, and instead fight tenaciously to the end. They may be disturbed by health proxies that constrain their options. Although experts as well as beginners hold this view, if there has been a shift in beliefs over time, it seems to have been in the direction of accepting death.

A priest made the same point: "When I first started in this business, I used to pray, let me just carry this person. Don't let him die. But then I realized, it's time for him to die. There's no place for him to go. No one wants to see a person that they've gotten close to and have a relationship with, die. But when you pull back and get rational about it, you ask yourself, 'What is the quality of life for this person going to be like?'" He went on to give the following illustration:

> There was Hector, on an oxygen mask in the hospital, gasping for a week. He [was near death but then] he had a rally. I walked into his room, and there he was; he'd ordered out for McDonald's chicken and was sitting there with drumsticks talking about going home. Well, while he was talking I had to think, home was a small room on 20th Street, and there

PRACTICAL TIPS FOR PHYSICIANS
LIMITING THE EFFECTS OF STRESS

(Obviously, no one can do all of the following. Even if you choose only one suggestion from each group, a difference in your stress level can be achieved. The point here is to exercise control over your professional life.)

Restructure Your Practice

- Close your practice to new patients for a period of time
- Add office staff, including other physicians, physician assistants, nurse practitioners

Change Your Scheduling Policy

- Build in time (20 to 30 minutes) for patient review, phone calls, and paperwork after several appointments
- Keep some time slots open every day for emergencies
- Make time to eat quietly

Participate in Non-Clinical Professional Activities

- Allot time for professional activities, e.g., conducting research, attending conferences, speaking on topics of interest
- Teach a course
- Consult (e.g., insurance companies, health care agencies)
- Serve on the board of a community-based AIDS organization
- Lecture at professional conferences and symposia
- Work with lobbying groups to effect change in AIDS policies and regulations

Get Away From It All

- Devote some specified time each week to a special interest or hobby (attend music concerts, films, or sports events; garden; do-it-yourself projects)
- Take several short holidays during the year (a 3- to 4-day weekend can be refreshing)
- Take a day-trip once a month with family or friends
- Spend an hour or two (lunch/dinner) with someone who is not a physician
- Change your daily routine and scenery occasionally (this can be done simply by taking another route to work)
- Sit down by yourself in a quiet room and rest

Exercise and Eat Well

- Take a walk two or three times a week
- Work out in a gymnasium or with a workout tape at home
- Participate in a sport (volleyball, swimming, basketball, tennis)
- Maintain consistent energy and health by eating a balanced diet and eating regularly

wasn't room for an oxygen tank, a home care worker, and Hector. So where could he go if this high was going to be maintained? There was no quality of life left for Hector. I wanted to believe [in his improvement] so bad that day, but when I left I had to think, "please God don't let it last because he's going to be one of the most miserable people in the world...."

The point of this story is not that poverty, in itself, disqualifies the value of living, but that in practice some circumstances may be so constricting that real quality of life is even further compromised.

The process of shifting gears involves practical, medical issues, as well as an emotional "letting go." For instance, shifting gears usually entails a significant change in the treatment plan. "I belonged to the hospice movement since the early eighties," one physician explained, "and that has helped me a lot with dealing with patients' deaths. That whole philosophy of death with dignity, free of pain, is a goal in itself. And I am not afraid of it."

Resistance or unwillingness to shift gears in end-stage illness can contribute to increased distress for both the patient and the physician. For example, one doctor said that the most emotionally exhausting aspect of his clinical work was "when I can't get someone out of the hospital, when there's nothing more I can do." His distress might be reduced if he were to perceive managing death as a challenge to be done well.

The process of "shifting gears" from active (at times aggressive, painful, and arduous) treatment to supportive or palliative care is complicated. Relevant considerations include timing of such a decision, doctor-patient communication, and patient (or proxy) consent. While this shift appears to be desirable, both physician and patient have to be ready. One physician explained, "If you don't let the patient know the time has come [for supportive care], you wind up doing a lot of unnecessarily cruel things to people." When the shift is successfully achieved, both physician and patient feel that the patient's wishes have been respected. (For more on this issue, see Chapter 11.)

Even the degree of palliative care offered varies from physician to physician. No doctor would withhold pain medication altogether, but some are more cautious in its use than others. For example, the amount of I.V. morphine they are willing to prescribe, and whether the dose schedule is fixed or flexible, may vary considerably. Few, if any, would discontinue anti-seizure medication or other symptom-controlling treatments until death appears imminent; decisions about use of compressed oxygen, transfusions, parenteral feeding, and hydration however, are more variable.

Many of these decisions depend to some extent on the availability of a written health proxy and the presence of the proxy in person. Although such documents tend to be less specific than most patients anticipate, some physicians will not act without written DNR ("do not resuscitate") orders. Others are comfortable doing so based on earlier conversations with the patient. Sometimes these decisions are complicated by the religious affiliation of a given hospital, although there is wide variation even within denominations. Two Catholic hospitals in the same community, for example, may have very different attitudes about such issues.

Overall, managing death effectively becomes an acceptable goal to physicians who conceptualize AIDS in terms of discrete stages, who acknowledge that there is a time for someone to die, and who recognize that at different stages, different strategies can be conducted well or poorly. Despite the reasonableness of these concepts, it is inevitable that physicians and other health care providers will, at times, feel great sadness, loss, and even anger. After detailing how she handles dying patients with great skill and sensitivity, one doctor concluded, "But there's just the sadness of caring for so many wonderful people who suffer. It's tragic, it's sad, and there's no way to make sense of it."

It's Okay to Cry, Sometimes

Caring for dying patients, especially those who are young, is an emotional business. A highly admired physician described an experience she had as an intern.

> When I met Gordon, he was in a coma from a drug overdose. My initial feelings toward him were very judgemental—if he tried to kill himself, why am I up in the middle of the night trying to rescue him? But when he came to, I learned that he was going blind, and he didn't want to be a burden to his friends, so he had tried to kill himself. Because he also had meningitis, he needed serial spinal taps. As I got to know him, he asked me to chat to distract him during the procedures. I eventually told him about a romantic relationship that was breaking up at that point. Soon after, he decided to go home to North Carolina, which was a brave thing to do because AIDS was new then. I went to say goodbye to him one afternoon, and as I sat on the edge of his bed, he said, "Well I hope things work out with your friend." I was overwhelmed by that. Here was this man who was dying and had gone blind and was going through this incredible journey, and he thought of my relationship and remembered what I'd said to him during a spinal tap. Tears just started flowing down my face. His mother saw them, but of course he couldn't have seen them. I kissed him goodbye and went out into the hall, and the whole sadness of his illness hit me, and his incredible generosity of heart. An attending physician who was working with me caring for another person tapped me on the shoulder. When I turned around and he saw that I was crying, he said, "It's okay, I'll talk to you some other time" and basically ran. Then the head nurse came up to me and gave me a big hug and said, "You really took good care of Gordon, and I know you're going to miss him." She just acknowledged that it was an emotional moment. She didn't say "Don't cry," or "Go ahead and cry." Just, "This is what's here." I was so grateful for that. And when I became a resident I really tried to help the students and interns talk about things of this sort.

Talking Things Out

While most physicians recognize the value of talking about and acknowledging feelings, in practice, it may be difficult for AIDS physicians to do so. It is widely believed that interacting with interested and friendly people is helpful to people experiencing difficult life circumstances. The types of support individuals seek in such situations and how they use them differ according to culture, class, ethnicity, gender, and age. Physicians, however, may be particularly reluctant to turn to others for solace, reassurance, and support during times of extreme stress.

Although some hospitals have organized support groups for their AIDS health workers, few physicians avail themselves of such services. There seems to be a sense among physicians that formal support groups are often not particularly useful or desirable. "We do have a support group that meets on a weekly basis," one doctor said, "but I think that day-by-day talking to colleagues about what's going on actually helps more. I mean you don't necessarily want to make a public announcement when you're feeling singularly inept. People connect more closely with one or two people than a whole group." Ironically, some physicians find that they cannot participate in a support group when they need it most. "I avoid it when I'm the most vulnerable," one doctor admitted, "and I attend when I'm the least vulnerable."

A priest engaged in AIDS ministry observed, "I would find it awkward to attend a support group that included other clergy with whom I'm dealing and working all the time. These are my peers. Letting them know where I'm vulnerable, how I may feel about a certain thing and what my weaknesses are, is a very touchy thing because I'm going to have to work with these people tomorrow. So where do I get support? A lot of us get it from within ourselves."

A West Coast physician initially attended a retreat organized for AIDS care providers with the intention of learning to better handle her patients' feelings. During the week, she realized, however, that

> This was about our feelings. What do you do when someone has a problem you can't fix? In school and during medical training you're taught, "You don't need to sleep, you don't need to eat, you don't need to rest. You don't need to be with your family." It's a horrible system. A lot of what I'm doing is un-learning. And, I'm learning to acknowledge that what we do is hard and that it's okay to feel overwhelmed, it's okay to feel sad, and it's okay not to like a patient.

Informal voluntary conversations with colleagues who are also friends appear to be helpful for some physicians, at least for certain kinds of problems. "If a patient's done something that I'm upset about, I schmooze with a colleague about it...and they'll understand how frustrated I feel. But if it's an emotional issue, like a patient's dying or I can't fix what's wrong or something like that, I don't deal with those issues well. I contain them. There are things I can't discuss."

Unfortunately, some physicians feel truly isolated in their work. "I'm not a good talker. There's nobody in my day-to-day life outside of this place who knows what it's like. You have to experience it to believe it. Who am I going to talk to? I don't have any friends. If I had a close friend, maybe that would be good. But how do you have the time?" This type of isolation may be a major by-product of overload that many AIDS physicians experience, if only transiently.

One physician study revealed that the solo AIDS practitioner experiences the most stress, particularly if he or she has minimal office staff, which, in a solo practice, is often the case.

Overall, it appears that physicians do not usually seek formal support groups. While most find it helpful to talk to colleagues about medical management issues, expressions of personal distress about their work are kept to a minimum. The implied elements of "therapy" and of personal exposure are not valued.

How Close Is Too Close?
There is striking disagreement about the appropriateness of personal closeness with patients among experienced AIDS specialists. Some physicians try to maintain more distance between themselves and their patients than they did in the past, to protect themselves. "I try not to really get too involved," one doctor explained. "I did that in the beginning, but you do so much hand-holding that you just wind up crying yourself. I don't get as friendly anymore because it's just too much. It's just too devastating to constantly lose friends."

Despite the potential for pain, other physicians are more apt to be emotionally connected to their patients, and they have no desire to change their natures. Furthermore, as people get very ill, it becomes difficult to maintain formalities. "You can be there when they need you, as long as they need you, and you can walk with them as far as they're going to go. Most of the time it is a privilege because you're learning from them and they're learning from you, and it's a give and take situation."

Emotional connectedness may be perceived as beneficial rather than costly for the health provider. "Yesterday, a former patient of mine came up the stairs just as I was getting ready to leave for lunch," one doctor recalled. "He said, 'Do you have a second?' And I answered, 'Well, just a second, but it's great to see you.' He had had to switch doctors because of insurance. And then he pulled out a bunch of flowers from behind his back and said, 'I really miss you.' That's what I think about when I wonder why I'm not burnt out. Even though this man could barely walk, he went across the street and got a bunch of flowers. He negotiated those stairs and asked me, 'Do you have a moment' to make sure he wasn't disturbing me. To me, that's a miracle."

Some physicians make home visits, either routinely or when "the patient is very ill, and there's nothing more I can do." Some have their home telephone numbers listed in the directory. Some go to funerals and memorial services, while others make it a policy never to do so. The choice of how close to get seems to be an individual one, without any clear advantage for one or another style for coping effectively.

BURNOUT

In some sense, "burnout" is the antithesis of the coping strategies just described. Although variously defined, the term "burnout" always refers to a state that is undesired and undesirable, regrettable, and involving an element of demoralization. Since the most systematic studies of burnout have been conducted by Maslach and Jackson (1981), we cite their definition: "Burnout is a situationally induced state characterized by emotional exhaustion which in turn leads to depersonalization (loss of empathy) and perceived (and often real) decline in personal accomplishment."

Another widely accepted notion of burnout is that it consists of an imbalance between giving and receiving, such that the person feels drained, without a sense of replenishment. A dramatic image of a literal burnout is offered by one observer: "In one way or another, we have all fashioned wings of feathers and wax and, like Icarus, flown too close to a symbolic sun and then plummeted emotionally" (Lynn, 1991). This reference to the myth of Icarus carries with it a central but often unacknowledged characteristic of burnout: it often befalls the most motivated and most eager.

Patients tell each other about doctors who appear to have reached a stage of burnout. They usually don't have time for patients. Burnt out physicians fail to return calls, routinely keep patients waiting for scheduled appointments, are rushed during the appointment, and no longer seem to have a personal interest. This is often considered the "price" of success. When young doctors enter practice and are well liked by their patients, the word spreads and their waiting rooms become crowded. Eventually they are overscheduled, with too many sick patients in the hospital, and don't have the time to be the humane, compassionate physicians that originally made them so attractive to patients.

Two points should be understood about burnout as a phenomenon. First, burnout should not be defined as the end result of overinvolvement or excessive emotional closeness per se. In our society, especially among males, any degree of emotionalism in a professional context is considered suspect. When we asked AIDS specialists about the degree of their emotional involvement with patients, a female physician responded emphatically, "When people say you're too involved it's like claiming you're too feminine. It becomes a negative quality. But being actively involved contributes a lot, I think, to the healing process." Decisions about whether to sit on the side of your patient's hospital bed or stand by it, whether or not to make house calls to homebound patients, or to attend funeral services are essentially a matter of personal style. While the level of emotional involvement certainly is related to the quality of fit between individual patients and physicians, it does not appear to be categorically good or bad, risky or not.

Second, the decision to stop working with patients who have HIV illness is not necessarily a reflection of burnout. The decision of AIDS doctors and nurses, or volunteers, to seek other kinds of work is not necessarily indicative of personal or systems failure. There may be times in a person's life when the nature of the work with PWAs (persons with AIDS) simply may or may not fit one's lifestyle. One of the most highly respected AIDS specialists we know had three children under the age of five. Moreover, her job and home were in different states. Between the demands of her work and the length of her daily commute, she often found herself in the supermarket at 10 P.M. at night. She eventually concluded that she didn't have the physical stamina to be both a good doctor and a good mother to small children. She left her position as chief of a major inpatient AIDS unit for a 9 to 5 job at an HMO near her home. She may make other professional changes as her children get older.

Burnout has been described as a "cop-out." One senior official of the American Medical Association refers to burnout as "a seductive concept...that gives you permission to leave the field of battle. But the patients and their families can't just walk away" (Jones, 1994). We don't agree. It may take particular grit to be an HIV care provider. This type of work may not be for everyone. "People who are dying and chronically ill require more of everything: time, energy, emotion," one physician noted. "That can be burdensome and some doctors really get tired of that. They want to go into a practice where they're not responsible for so much." It is far better to "leave the field" than to remain feeling demoralized, harassed, and pessimistic.

Those who work with PWAs risk singeing their wings when they seek the impossible. As one physician recalled, "I had this whole Mother Teresa thing. I'd work til 10 P.M. every night and weekends. When I'd talk to friends who aren't health care workers, they'd tell me I'm a lunatic and urged me to get real. So I put Mother Teresa back in the closet and learned to take time off."

Some physicians understand the road to burnout and its consequences but seem powerless to prevent it. "I'm chronically on the edge of burnout, if I'm not in it. It is a sense of exhaustion, feeling overwhelmed, feeling distant, almost a lack of concern. When it's bad, there is forgetfulness, memory loss, making mistakes, and certainly a loss of humor. For me, it stems from a lack of collegiality, of not having partners to talk to. I think having colleagues in the office with whom to share the burden and to discuss things would be a relief. But I'm a loner. For me, in solo practice, it's the frustration of not having the time to manage my business and my staff, because I have to take care of patients who are always my primary responsibility."

Preventing burnout is usually a matter of how a health professional takes care of him or herself. Arranging adequate coverage and time off appear to be helpful strategies.

Dealing with Illness Progression and Death
Some AIDS specialists acknowledge being upset by their inability to cure

patients and by their ultimate deaths, while others indicate that death, in general, does not cause significant distress. These physicians are referring to patient deaths that are expected, deaths that come after a gradual, worsening course of illness.

The unanticipated death is almost invariably troubling. "Death usually doesn't bother me," one doctor explained, "except when I'm surprised." It is emotionally draining when, unexpectedly, "the patient develops a brutal and rapidly fatal form of this disease." At least two factors appear to contribute to this fairly universal source of distress. The first is simply the suddenness of the event—the physician has had no time to prepare. Another source of pain in the "premature" or unexpected death is the implication that the physician is somehow culpable.

Physicians also feel more distress when a clustering of deaths occurs all at once, in contrast to the "ordinary" rate of loss. Unfortunately, this simply happens from time to time in the life of an AIDS physician.

Special Relationships

The loss of a particular patient may also cause more distress than the loss of the average patient. Sometimes the death of a "really very young patient is very hard." More generally, there are just some patients who become "special" and whose loss is especially distressing. "There are particular patients one gets really attached to...often these people become very close to me and it's definitely more difficult when you run into trouble with them." The loss of physician-patients also tends to be particularly emotionally exhausting.

Another difficult loss, and one that may be unique to AIDS medicine, is the loss of friends one's own age. This is particularly true for younger gay physicians who accept their friends as patients, in contrast to those who become friendly with people only after they become patients.

The heartbreak of deterioration is much more intense for the physician if the patient was known to him or her when he was still well. In contrast, consultants haven't witnessed decline. An infectious disease consultant who rarely provided primary care, for example, observed, "The first person I actually diagnosed with *Pneumocystis* was a musician, and I saw him in the hospital when he was quite ill. There was a poster on the bulletin board in his room about his records, but I didn't recognize the face. I looked at the poster and asked, 'Who's that?' He said, 'That's me.' I didn't recognize him. The photo on the poster was of a person who was well."

Often the death of a "long-term survivor" is especially troubling because of the duration of the relationship, the physician's pride in how well the patient had been doing, the number of past crises that had been weathered together, and the attachments of office staff. At least part of the distress might be attributed to the magical belief in the literal meaning of long-term survivor—here was someone who might really make it.

Overall, nearly all experienced AIDS physicians are able to handle most patient deaths without severe distress. Nevertheless, unanticipated deaths, or the loss of specific patients are bound to be troubling. The bottom line is that no matter how experienced physicians are or how many deaths they encounter, there will always be particular losses that will be more difficult than others.

Gay Doctors, Straight Doctors
The HIV specialist who is gay must sooner or later address the implications of risk-group membership. As one noted, "It's one thing to work in the arena of HIV health care. It's another to be a member of a high-risk group yourself. You have to deal with the whole concept of survivor guilt. I've seen some people push themselves, partially for that reason. There are very different psychological burdens [for gay and straight AIDS specialists]. Doctors who don't belong to the community don't necessarily see themselves as the patient or the lover."

On the other hand, gay physicians may be able to draw on unique sources of gratification in their work. As a female AIDS specialist observed, "I think the stress of HIV work on some levels is balanced for many of us, particularly gay and lesbian doctors, because we are caring for our community." Another reward is recognition and respect within the gay community, which is intensified in cities with strongly delineated gay neighborhoods. "When I go out to get a loaf of bread on my street, often I meet someone who cares about someone I'm treating. And that's really nice. It's a real sense of connectedness." People also seem to recognize the increasing burdens on HIV doctors, and that, in an indirect way, is also very supportive.

Heterosexual doctors also face risks and challenges as AIDS specialists. A gay physician pointed out, "A lot of people I work with very closely are not gay. I know of one physician, for example, whose wife is not very supportive of her husband's practice, and has been pressuring him for years: 'Get out of this, you're putting me at risk, you're putting our children at risk, you don't have to do this.' Straight doctors may not have the support structures that I do." Thus, while physicians who are themselves members of the gay community may be subject to unique stressors, they may also benefit from unique buffers. On balance, there appear to be no differences between gay and "straight" practitioners in terms of dedication, perceived stress, or likelihood of leaving AIDS medicine.

Physicians Are Human, Too
It may be not so much the volume of work, which can be controlled, as the "sense of relentlessness" that eventually takes a heavy toll. The pressures of treating serious illness and dealing with multiple deaths are common sources of ongoing stress for physicians. "On a given day," one physician lamented, "it may seem just like a march, one after the other. On a bad day, everyone's sick." Another explained, "I've come to accept a white blood count of 1.5 as normal. In a lot of these patients, every single laboratory value is abnormal. What the hell do you do? Following these people, unless you have a real

shell, can make you crazy...you hurt afterwards. And the patient population turns over fully every 3 years."

One physician addressed the specific problem of too many medical exigencies:

> It starts from the minute I strap on the beeper in the morning to the time I go to bed, and many times I can't sleep through the night without a phone call. Today, I've got a guy in the Emergency Room, another guy in the Holding Area, another guy going for surgery. I've got to rush in and discharge two patients today. I've got to call orders to the home care company. I've got to see twenty-five patients in the office. I've got a ton of paperwork. I've got a desk I haven't seen the top of in God knows how long. I want to write a book but how in hell am I going to write a book? How am I going to do my consulting work? I have a conference to prepare for. And I haven't seen my kids awake in 3 days.

This man leaves the house before 8 A.M. and returns between 9 P.M. and midnight.

Another physician noted, "The most difficult times are when I feel overwhelmed, when I have too many sick people at one time, which you can't control, when the hospital is full of patients—maybe eight or ten people in the hospital—and an office filled with sick patients. To me that's the very worst."

Despite the emotional toll, of the physicians we interviewed, nearly all planned to continue to practice as AIDS specialists, barring major changes in the reimbursement structure. A few expressed the need for help or a wish to retire in 10 years. The others envisioned continuing their work until "the epidemic ends."

REFERENCES

Lynn R. Burnout and the professional care giver. In: Haworth Press, 1989, pp. 21-26. Cited in *AIDS Reader: Burnout in healthcare and support in relation to HIV and AIDS*. Nationale Commissie AIDS Bestrijing, September 1991.

Maslach C, Jackson SE. The measurement of experienced burnout. *Journal of Occupational Behavior*. 1981;2;99-13.

Jones L. Will attention bring action? *American Medical News*. 1994; Jan 17:1,33.

10

LIVING WITH PROLONGED ILLNESS: PATIENTS' REACTIONS AND STRATEGIES

COMMENT

In the context of AIDS, the conventional notion of hope may require modification. The standard scale used to measure hope in psychiatric research (Beck, 1974) begins by asking the respondent to agree or disagree with the statement: "I look forward to the future with hope and enthusiasm." People who are clinically depressed almost invariably score this item as "false," whereas people who see themselves and want others to see them as upbeat and positive score it as "true," even when they have late-stage HIV illness, including two or three incurable infections. The men and women quoted in this chapter value themselves enough to struggle daily with complex medical regimens intended to extend their lives. Yet they really don't "look forward to the future with hope and enthusiasm" in the conventional sense. "Hope" in this context refers to the idea that there continues to be value in being alive and that there is more to learn, to experience, and to accomplish, even in the presence of physical limitations and the anticipation of progressive decline.

As duration and patterns of HIV illness have changed over the past decade, so has the experience of living with AIDS. In this chapter, a range of survival strategies is illustrated by seven people who candidly describe their reactions to living with protracted illness.

LIVING IN A CHANGING EPIDEMIC

Living with AIDS is a tremendously complicated and variable experience. The particular viral strain involved; the person's genetic makeup and personal, medical, and social resources; as well as simple luck all affect the patient's medical course, outlook, and expectations. In addition, the type of initial diagnosis and subsequent infections determine the balance between periods of relative health and episodes of illness. Over the past decade, changes in many of these variables have altered the experience and expectations of people with HIV illness.

Changes in Illness Patterns

The onset and type of initial AIDS-defining condition are changing. In 1982 and 1983, the diagnoses of *Pneumocystis carinii* pneumonia (PCP) and Kaposi's sarcoma (KS) were the most common AIDS-defining conditions, and PCP was often fatal during the first or second illness episode. Because of successful prophylactic and treatment interventions, PCP is no longer a commonly lethal initial AIDS-defining illness. For reasons not well understood, KS occurs now less often as an initial diagnosis, at least in the United States (Weiss et al, 1993). PCP as an initial diagnosis declined in one large study from 57% before 1986 to 31% in the years from 1988 to 1993 (Osmond et al, 1994). During this same period, initial diagnoses of chronic and often incurable opportunistic infections such as cytomegalovirus (CMV) and *Mycobacterium avium intracellulare* (also known as MAI), increased substantially (Hoover et al, 1993).

Changes in Survival Time

Duration of survival after initial clinical AIDS diagnosis has also changed, creating a "generational" effect. During the 1980s, development of effective treatment and prophylaxis of acute PCP meant that the initial episode of an opportunistic infection was postponed until later in the course of HIV illness. Now, when people do eventually have an acute illness, the immune system is often more compromised and the T cell count is lower.

In longitudinal studies of two cohorts of gay men followed from 1983 to 1993, Osmond and colleagues (1994) concluded that "the shift toward diagnoses with poor prognosis worked against larger overall improvement in survival time from [clinical] AIDS to death" (p 1084). Overall, they found "little increase in time from clinical AIDS to death but a significant increase of about 1 year in survival time from a CD4 lymphocyte count [of 200 or less] to death between October 1983 and November 1986, and the November 1986 to November 1988 period." That is, a growing number of people with very low T cells remain healthy longer than in the past. No subsequent improvement was found between 1988 and 1993, although data for this follow-up period are incomplete. Some improvement in time from clinical diagnosis to death was found for patients whose initial diagnosis was PCP or KS, but not other diagnoses, a finding confirmed by a report of over 6,000 patients in 17 European countries between 1979 and 1989.

These decade-long longitudinal studies were begun when the only populations recognized to be disproportionately infected were gay men, and, in smaller numbers but even greater percent, hemophiliacs. Much less is known about the longitudinal course of illness in HIV-infected drug users and women. Because these two groups tend to have fewer social and financial resources, their access and utilization of medical care may be more limited. Therefore, the course and expression of illness over time for the latter groups may be somewhat different from those of the former.

Changes in Expectations

Despite the absence of known effective treatments in the early and middle 1980s, people first diagnosed in these years often believed that their task was to "buy time," to hold on and stay alive until there was a breakthrough (at least stabilization if not cure), which was seen as imminent. Today, many of these surviving patients with AIDS (PWAs), as well as many who are newly diagnosed with an AIDS-defining condition, no longer expect a breakthrough to occur in their lifetimes. Most think it will occur, if at all, years from now, not in time for them.

This change in perspective was expressed by a surviving partner talking shortly after his lover's death:

> After R's initial illness in 1987, we made plans. He bounced back very strongly from his initial PCP, and we formulated a really good plan for the future. We really thought we'd get to it. We thought, *surely*, if he could last 2 years, there'd be a treatment. There'd be *something* that would help you to be stable; maybe you'd always live with jeopardized health, but you'd be able to live your life. We really thought that. In June 1987, a lot of people thought that. Who'd have imagined how little progress would be made in all these years! There's so little hope in the articles these days talking about the 10-year anniversary [of the identification of AIDS].

Reactions to Living with AIDS

Below are voices of long-term survivors, interviewed between 1990 and 1993, some on several occasions. What we consider an essential element in these statements is the candid and unwincing articulation of the harsh realities of living with AIDS superimposed on both verbal and behavioral affirmations of hope and intent to survive. To be so forthright about one's fears and doubts is seldom encouraged or rewarded in our society. These selections illustrate different ways of living with AIDS.

John

A 50-year-old minister, John was diagnosed with PCP in 1987. In 1992, he was taking 43 HIV pills a day. Although not hospitalized since 1988, he has had a variety of debilitating constitutional symptoms (e.g., prolonged bouts of fever, episodic nausea, chronic pain from neuropathy) and illnesses (e.g., tuberculosis).

> We were saying in '87, '88, '89 that we were buying time until there was a breakthrough. Now we know there won't be one in our lifetimes. All of this is a hypothetical thing for us. And then there is the stress of living with this, the stress of every day knowing you are getting closer to the end. You see yourself fail, just a little bit more, just a nuance maybe, but there is a

lessening of something in you. You realize that more and more of you isn't working. And more and more of you is dying. It used to be, "Wow, I'm still alive, and I feel good." Over time, it's "Wow, I am still alive and look at how much I have lost, and what more will be asked of me tomorrow?"

I think when you're just diagnosed you think you're going to beat this. You don't quite understand the disease. You don't quite understand the odds. You don't quite understand what you just heard. You think, "It's not going to happen to me." And then as you go along and your friends start getting sick and dying and you start getting sicker, you see the same road they were on and you know you're not going to beat it. Sometimes you're very uncertain how you're going to deal with it—if you even want to continue dealing with it.

Some people take the attitude, "I'm going to make a statement. I'm going to handle this well. I can deal." And those very people after a while start thinking, "Make a statement to whom? Who cares?" And it doesn't seem like anyone does care. You're in the middle of a plague. There are a lot of people trying to make the same statement and you're just one of a crowd, but nobody's listening.

When you start out, you've got friends, you've got support. One of the saddest things is the loneliness of being a long-term survivor. Your friends are gone, your address book is thin; there's nobody left that you used to know and depend on. And this happens when you're getting sick and it's harder to get out and meet people, even if you want to.

Richard

A 34-year old writer and arts critic, Richard had also hoped to be an actor. He experienced his first episode of PCP in July 1986. At that time, his CD4 count was under 50. He regained his health and devoted his considerable energies and abilities to being an AIDS activist. He remained relatively well until 1989 when he began daily infusions of ganciclovir (Cytovene) for CMV colitis. In April 1990, he developed CMV retinitis, and foscarnet (Foscavir) was added to his infusion regimen. He was hospitalized between 1989 and 1990 more than 15 times, but not at all in 1991. His vision remained largely intact until about 6 months before his death in July 1992. When asked about living with AIDS in 1991, these were his thoughts:

> I've wanted to write about living with AIDS as opposed to just dying from it because it seems like more and more people are going to live quite a long time with it. That's a whole different situation from the old days when you just died very quickly. Since I've been sick now for almost 5 years, it's become a way of life, not just an automatic death, and that's a different range of experiences. It would be a lot easier just to die quickly than live year after year with constant chronic illness. It's much slower, much more measured, and in a way much more difficult. It's not as dramatic, and the ups and downs are not as constant, but the patience required is much

more taxing in a way that requires adjusting to a completely new way of life.

There seems to be very little pleasure in terms of the old kind of pleasure that we're accustomed to. Eating has become very difficult for me. Sexual activity is at a very low level, partly because of physical limitations and partly because of a loss of interest. In terms of physical things, the only pleasure I have is lying down. I guess pleasure has become more cerebral for me. But even what used to bring intense pleasure has its shadow now.

As the years go by, more and more I think my friends and family are pulling me along—reluctantly. A lot of them are literally propping me up, pulling me through this, dragging me along. A lot of times when I feel I can't go on for myself any more, I feel I should go on for them.

As the years go by, you ask yourself, "How many years of this can I have, of really being an invalid?" It's like being a child again and everyone else is out playing, and you have to stay home and do your homework, forever.

After almost 5 years, I've nearly run out of personal resources. It comes back to the question of looking at the future and seeing years of being an invalid. Is it worth it? I think I hear from a lot of people with AIDS that the prospect of dying is not as scary as the prospect of years and years and years of living with this.

Charlie

After giving up a potentially brilliant academic or government career in foreign relations, Charlie had been a writer and editor. He decided that pursuing his PhD and a career in the State Department were incompatible with a radical gay lifestyle. In 1981, he was told that he had gay related immune deficiency (GRID). Since 1984 he has had recurrent illnesses, but was formally diagnosed with an AIDS condition (PCP) only in 1987. In 1989, MAI was diagnosed. He also had severe neuropathy, which impaired his mobility and interfered with bladder control. In reflecting about the effect of AIDS on his life he declared:

I've lasted quite some time with a very damaged immune system because I have the heart of a lion, but this disease has absolutely crushed me. It is the most monstrous thing I can imagine ever happening. I have not reconciled myself one bit to it. I'm in a state of shock to this day that something so awful could happen. I have unbelievable pain and rage. AIDS has put a huge dagger through my life, essentially cutting my life in half. I would have to say that there is nothing that has eased the difficulty and emotional pain of this situation. As far as I am concerned, my life ended in June of 1987. I feel an underlying terror dating from that day which has never waned at all.

But my tenacious life force has been there right from the beginning. You find out about yourself when you're in a crisis, and the things I've found out about myself are good. No matter how much I've struggled mentally and physically, I have shown a tremendous fighting spirit and everyone around me sees it, and knows it and that's something that I'm proud of. I know what I'm up against and every day it requires strategic choices, but I work with my doctor and I make my decisions. I've been isolated for quite some time, but now I'm out a bit more, seeing other PWAs, and I'm learning a lot about what courage is all about and where it is in me.

Realizing that we have low points and coming back from them doesn't relieve the fear and that crushed feeling. It utterly crushed my life and the pieces are all over the floor. Can I cope with this or not? That's what it comes down to. It doesn't get easier. It gets harder. I just question how long I can continue to cope.

Iris

It is hard for Iris even to describe herself: "I have experienced such behavioral extremes in one lifetime that I don't really know who the fuck I am. I'm a court-reporter/rock-star/drug addict," which is as good a description as any. She grew up in the homes of various relatives, foster parents, and mental institutions, ran away at age 15, and became a serious heroin addict. She says that she was aware of AIDS as a phenomenon in general and as a personal disaster long before most professionals. She tells her story,

Back in 1981, maybe 1980, I was seeing something very weird. I was addicted to heroin, and I was in a medical detox unit where they give you methadone whether you want it or not. They had a guy up there who had been thrown out of prison because they wouldn't feed him; people were terrified. He got sick inside [in prison], and they put him in the Beth Israel ward, and he was dying of AIDS. He was a young guy, in his thirties. And he said, "I don't know what the fuck is going on. I don't know what I've got." And maybe 6 months later I was in the hospital again, and another guy was up there that I knew as a dope fiend, even younger than the first. He was in his twenties—he died on his birthday. They wouldn't even take the food trays from his room. When they walked down the hall, the nurses were covered from head to foot in these huge helmets and these gowns that went all the way down to their ankles, and even their feet were covered in bags with drawstrings. It was still called GRID [gay related immune deficiency], and they said only gay people got it. All of a sudden, there was a rash of deaths among hypodermic drug users. Most of those people were so out of it, they didn't think anything of it. But I noticed it right away. When I saw the first guy I said, "Motherfucker." "Thanks a lot God." I knew. I said, "If he's got it, we've *all* got it. We've all got it."

A drug addict has two diseases to worry about. They got AIDS, and they got another disease. If they don't remember that disease, that addiction will kill them in such a fast and vicious way that they won't have the opportunity to die comfortably in some nice clean hospital with AIDS. They'll die like an animal, and somebody will throw their body in a dumpster or any place they can get rid of it, and that's what a junkie's death is.

When asked whether she ever feels like giving up, Iris answered: "A couple of times. But I always feel like getting high. That's the dope fiend's national anthem. That's the equivalent of a square person saying, 'I'm going to kill myself.'" But Iris has come to terms in this way:

> I've been more depressed than most people have ever experienced. I have even been in a couple of really black spaces spiritually, and survived it. I'm not afraid of depression; I'm not afraid of looking at those phantoms. I believe in God. I think that loss of faith is the root of depression. Life is hard, and it is painful, and we all go through these terrible abandonments. But life is also a spiritual trip, and when I realized that, I lost my desire to destroy myself. Something happened to me when I quit using drugs: I began to realize that life and being alive was the greatest, most unbelievable gift that anybody could ever have. Not whether you're rich or poor, whether you're crippled or blind, or whether you have AIDS or you don't have AIDS. Life is an opportunity to know God. And to throw that away is a real tragedy.

Iris is now determined to finish the training she once started as a court stenographer; her life and her outlook can fairly be described as utterly transformed.

Mitchell

A very visible public figure, Mitchell was diagnosed in 1982 with what later was classified as an AIDS-defining condition. Despite six hospitalizations and recurrent bouts of pneumonia, diarrhea, and KS, he continued to write, travel, and speak in the United States and abroad. His death after Christmas in 1993 shocked the HIV community because he had seemed to be truly an AIDS "survivor" in the unusual sense of the word.

> I think the single most important reason I've lived all these years with AIDS has been the accident of my doctor, specifically the PCP prophylaxis that he started in 1983. Thanks to him, I came to AIDS very Western, very pill oriented. I would have jumped on many a bandwagon, but he always talked me out of it. I have to understand the theoretical mechanisms by which something is supposed to work, and if it can't be explained to me I generally don't bother. Now I'm prophylaxing against five major OIs [opportunistic infections] that kill us. Of course, there haven't been studies proving that these medications actually prevent the OIs, but I think a case can be made.
>
> I tolerate the drugs well, so I feel that I'm buying time. But I guess I feel rationally that AIDS will get me. I don't know when, but it will get me. The way I choose to process that is that it's almost a blessing to know how your end is going to come, if not when. I was on a plane that almost crashed—wind shear—and the pilot tried to make two landings. I was cool

as a cucumber. I knew I would not die in a plane crash. That's not how I'm going to go.

I don't like taking all the pills, doing all the medical routines. I sometimes joke that I'm ready for the next epidemic; I'm tired of this one. I would like to have a day where I don't think about it or talk about it.

I think part of the reason I still feel good is that prior to AIDS my life was full of regret, things I wished I'd done differently. But there isn't much in the last 8 years I regret or that I would change, which is not the same thing as saying I didn't make major mistakes. My missions have been very clear. I often say that if I die tomorrow, I will have lived a full life. I consider that a really precious gift. I don't want to die tomorrow. I've got a lot more plans and living to do, but I feel I've had an impact, I guess.

I'm completely different than I was prior to getting sick. I'm much more who I always wanted to be. Who I always imagined I would be. I just didn't know when to begin getting serious about it. AIDS made that very clear. It made me serious about every aspect of my life. I think at 26 you're entitled to be a little silly and not be into grand-scheme, long-term kinds of things, but AIDS smacks that out of you.

Another important thing is to go through your depression and really have it. The New Age terminology is to really experience your death and then get on with living. You ask, "What is the worst case scenario?" And then you prepare yourself. When some version of that happens, you feel you've been there before and can handle it. You live one day at a time. You might wake up one day and discover you're 10 years down the road.

In the last published interview before he died, Mitchell meditated about his approaching death.

I once gave a glib quote. At the end of *The Plague*, Camus says that, ultimately, plague teaches us that there's more in mankind to admire than despise. I used to say that what this plague has taught me is that it's a dead heat. They are absolutely neck and neck. But I would say now, as I end my life, Camus was right. That which is good is better than that which is bad. That which is good is worth enduring the bad for. In my life, the suffering and pain and horror and atrocity have been more than balanced out by the joy.

Rachel
A 50-year-old health professional who found out she was HIV-positive in 1986, Rachel developed lymphoma in 1991. She was successfully treated, and the lymphoma is now in remission. In talking about her life with HIV, she mused:

The diagnosis of lymphoma was certainly a jolt to my ego. I don't know why I thought somehow that everyone else was going to die and I was going to remain alive. When I was diagnosed with lymphoma, it really shook me. It was like, cancer and AIDS, excuse me! And I wasn't at all sure what treatments I wanted, or even if I wanted them, and I still go through that.

There were times, there still are times, when I think it isn't worth struggling. But I show up for my life! Sometimes it feels like, "Oh, shit! I have to make another decision about my health, or it's another doctor, or it's another...." And it's further complicated because a lot of my friends have passed away. I feel I'm developing a certain numbness about that, which is fine. Often I feel I have to keep moving. It's like that feeling inside of not stopping to feel grief. And I have pain, now, too. Sometimes when the body hurts, you get real confused about what's going on. But there's a lot of things that interest me. I've been very involved with groups and workshops. I'd like to write a book for women who have been in recovery dealing with HIV. Maybe do some floral arranging, something different. And continue my rewarding relationship.

There are people in my life who love me and whom I love. There's a support system I can relate to and enjoy. I have a working relationship with my doctors, and I really know what I want to do with my own health care, no matter what the outcome is. I love the AIDS community. I have love in my life and goals.

Josh

Trained in the fine arts and acting, Josh was working as an administrator at a social agency when interviewed. He also had had a life-threatening illness with initial full recovery. His first AIDS-defining condition was lymphoma, which was found in the bone marrow. While undergoing aggressive chemotherapy, he developed a blood clot in the brain. Both the lymphoma and the clot were successfully treated during a 3-month period, and he has been in remission since then, working full-time as director of a community AIDS organization.

> People with AIDS get so sick and yet keep coming back. It's an amazing thing to see. But when the peaks over time get lower and lower, and the valleys predominate, then the picture changes. I had a horrible illness that was life threatening; and I did chemo, I lost my hair, I threw up constantly. But in 3 months it was over. I was well, sick and well again. That's very different from living day to day with fatigue, with low-grade fever, or with mild nausea that doesn't go away. That's wearing. It can cause exhaustion. For me, after surviving the lymphoma and being declared in remission, I realized, "Holy shit, I'm not going to die. I'm still here and I have to get on with my life." I left a bad relationship; I got my own apartment for the first time. I now make more money than I ever did, and I'm fighting to stay alive and live my life.

Two years later, Josh is alive, well, and very active in an agency serving the needs of PWAs.

COPING STRATEGIES OF PWAS

Living with HIV disease is a psychological as well as medical challenge.

Effective patients are usually those who remain active about fighting their illness (at least until they deliberately choose to stop fighting, a subject discussed in Chapter 11). When asked what advice they would give someone who is newly diagnosed, many long-term survivors said, "Maintain a positive attitude; don't think of it as a death sentence." This advice can be quite difficult to follow, however, when one sees so many friends die. The task then becomes not to give up and to remain active in managing one's health and life while being realistic about the medical requirements of the disease. In this context, the "Alcoholics Anonymous Prayer" is apt: "God grant me the serenity to accept the things I cannot change, the courage to change the things I can, and the wisdom to know the difference."

With HIV disease, it is difficult for patients to know what they and their physicians have control over and can change. The person with HIV must learn to live with uncertainty about the future and the course of disease progression, if not the outcome. The people interviewed for this book, both doctors and patients, have described certain characteristics associated with doing better under these difficult circumstances.

Stress and Coping: Jargon Translated

According to a widely held psychological theory, developed by Lazarus and Folkman (1984), a stressful situation is considered to be "personally significant to one's well-being while taxing or exceeding one's resources. The psychological distress of stressful situations is modified by two processes: situational appraisals of control, and coping." The term, "situational appraisals of control" refers to the extent that one believes a situation can be managed or changed. Coping is defined as "thoughts and behaviors that the person uses to manage or alter the problem that is causing distress (problem-focused coping) and regulate the emotional response to the problem (emotion-focused coping)" (Folkman et al, 1993). Emotion-focused coping strategies (including avoidance, keeping one's feelings to oneself, seeking emotional support, reappraising the situation in a positive light) predominate when the person perceives less control over the source of distress.

Recent research with long-term AIDS survivors (Remien et al, 1992) has investigated ways of coping with protracted illness as well as extended and unanticipated survival following an AIDS diagnosis among 53 gay men interviewed in 1990 and 1991. No single coping style emerged as contributing to positive survival; rather, the long-term survivors made use of numerous methods, such as taking personal action with regard to medical care, re-evaluating and modifying goals and relationships, community involvement, and pursuing enjoyable activities.

Are Avoidance and Denial Necessarily Bad?

The adaptive values of a positive attitude, a fighting spirit, a confrontational orientation to AIDS have been emphasized throughout this book for their impact on mental health and its potential effect on prolonging survival. There is the possibility, however, that the converse may be true; that for some individuals, refusal to acknowledge what is probably "true" may also be effective.

In the scientific literature, "active" coping is commonly associated with better psychological outcome than "avoidant" coping. This has been reported for patients with cancer and other illnesses, as well as those with HIV infection (see Remien et al, 1992, for a review of this literature). Similar assumptions are found in the traditional literature on "positive mental health," defined as an accurate perception of reality without distortions to meet one's wishes (Jahoda, 1958). Kubler-Ross, in her widely read book, *On Death and Dying*, writes that "acceptance" is the final stage in adjustment to terminal illness, a stage "almost devoid of feelings," where the patient "will have mourned the impending loss of so many meaningful people and places and he will contemplate his coming end with a certain degree of quiet expectation" (1969, p 112).

The concept of "denial," which derives from psychoanalytic theory about defense mechanisms, has had a negative reputation since Freud's day. According to a well-known psychologist, all defense mechanisms "disclosed by psychoanalytic study are for the most part somewhat primitive ways of coping with danger. They are not ideal solutions; they all imply that the true state of affairs has been somewhat falsified in the interests of safety. This is most evident in what is probably the most primitive of the mechanisms, *denial....*" (White, 1952, p 314).

There is another body of psychological research that leads to quite different conclusions. Taylor and colleagues (1988) have conducted a series of studies showing that "rather than being characterized by realistic perceptions, normal human perception is characterized by unrealistic optimism about the future, an exaggerated sense of personal control, and self-aggrandizing self-perceptions." These "positive illusions" were related to traditional criteria for mental health; in their research, those who were identified as clinically depressed actually had more realistic perceptions than those considered mentally healthy.

More recently, Taylor and colleagues (1992) have studied the attitudes and health status of HIV seropositive gay men with absent to mild symptoms. In keeping with their earlier findings, men with unrealistically optimistic beliefs about the probable course of HIV illness were considered to have better psychological adjustment or to be engaged in more active coping. The converse also was shown in a sample of 74 men with AIDS (Reed et al, in press, 1994). High scores on a brief pencil and paper measure of "realistic acceptance" of their risk for future debilitation and mortality were associated with *decreased* survival time. This relationship held even when the investigators controlled for other psychological factors, such as depression, and physical factors, such as disease status and level of energy. "Realistic acceptance" is viewed by these investigators as a coping strategy but seems more accurately identified as a form of situational appraisal, to use the Lazarus and Folkman (1984) distinction.

It seems likely that the adaptive value of realistic perception and confrontation, versus unrealistic optimism and denial, may be related to an individual's time and place in life. In a literal sense, the odds of living one's full life span after a diagnosis of HIV illness are certainly reduced. Some would say it is not even a matter of odds, which implies a degree of uncertainty about outcome. The positive attitude that is so widely praised by doctors and patients alike almost always entails some degree of "unrealistic" appraisal of the future or some distortion of probabilities. Certainly the man with a CD4 cell count of 20 who describes his health needs as "those of a typical 50-year-old man who happens to be HIV positive" and who has never consulted an HIV specialist is not promoting optimal care for himself. On the other hand, the person who concludes that he has 3 months left to live because that is the median survival reported for a given diagnosis in a medical journal, and who, therefore, plans to use up his resources in that time frame, is also not acting wisely.

We think it is useful to consider both *adaptive* and *malignant* avoidance and denial. What is adaptive and what is malignant depends to some extent on timing, circumstance, and the magnitude of the alterations in perception or understanding that denial implies.

REFERENCES

Beck A, Weissman A, Lester D, et al. The measure of pessimism: the Hopelessness Scale. *Journal of Consulting and Clinical Psychology*. 1974;42:861-865.

Folkman S, Chesney M, Pollack L, Coates T. Stress, control, coping and depressive mood in HIV-positive and -negative gay men in San Francisco. *Journal of Nervous and Mental Disease*. 1993; 181:409-416.

Hoover DR, Saah A, Bacellar H, et al. Clinical manifestations of AIDS in the era of pneumocystis prophylaxis. *New England Journal of Medicine*. 1993;329:1922-1926.

Jahoda M. *Current Concepts of Positive Mental Health*. New York: Basic Books; 1958.

Kubler-Ross E. *On Death and Dying*. New York: Macmillan; 1969.

Lazarus R, Folkman S. *Stress, Appraisal and Coping*. New York: Springer; 1984.

Osmond D, Charlebois E, Lang W, et al. Changes in AIDS survival time in two San Francisco cohorts of homosexual men, 1983 to 1993. *Journal of the American Medical Association*. 1994;271:1083-1087.

Reed G, Kemeny M, Taylor S, et al. 'Realistic acceptance' as a predictor of psychological adjustment and survival time in gay men with AIDS. *Health Psychology*. In press.

Remien RH, Rabkin JG, Williams J, Katoff L. Coping strategies and health beliefs of AIDS longterm survivors. *Psychology and Health*. 1992;6:335-345.

Taylor SE, Brown JD. Illusion and well-being: a social psychological perspective on mental health. *Psychological Bulletin* 1988;103:193-210.

Taylor SE, Kemeny M, Aspinwall L, et al. Optimism, coping, psychological distress, and high-risk sexual behavior among men at risk for AIDS. *Journal of Personality and Social Psychology.* 1992;63:460-473.

Weiss P, Wallace M, Olson P, et al. Changes in the mix of AIDS-defining conditions (letter). *New England Journal of Medicine.* 1993;329:1962.

White W. *Lives in Progress.* New York: Dryden Press; 1952.

11

THE END OF THE LINE FOR PWAS: WHEN ENOUGH IS ENOUGH

COMMENT

Some patients, at some time late in their illnesses, choose to determine the timing of their deaths. Sometimes this decision entails the discontinuation of treatments that may still have some therapeutic effect. In other cases, it may mean taking pills or starting intravenous morphine with the intention of its "double effect:" relieving pain and accelerating an inevitable and impending death. The latter options clearly are more accessible at home than in the hospital, where legal constraints are more salient, and where private initiative is often not feasible. It appears that knowledge that they have the right—and the means—to determine the time of their deaths often helps to sustain people and to extend the duration of their willingness to live.

"If never good, if sometime, why not now?" This question was asked in the fourth century by a terminally ill bishop when urged by Augustine to stave off death a little longer. (Augustine is said to have admired this response.) It represents an acknowledgement of choice about when to die that is a recurrent theme in Western culture. It is only in recent times, however, that biomedical advances have allowed mechanical postponement of death and raised legal issues regarding who is entitled to choose the timing of death.

Although there is a wealth of excellent writing by social historians, ethicists, medical sociologists, and other academicians concerned with the nature of death in contemporary society, these discussions tend to be general (Madan, 1992; Aries, 1981; Hamel, 1991; Hastings Center, 1992) or to address specific cases (Dworkin, 1991; Wolf, 1990). Issues concerning physician-assisted suicide have received exceptionally thoughtful and reasoned consideration in leading medical journals during the past decade (Quill et al, 1992; Brody, 1992; Miskin, 1991; Wanzer et al, 1989). These discussions address germane issues although they also refer to the general

This chapter has been expanded with permission from a previously published article in *PAACNOTES* (January 1993:24-27, 46-47).

class of very ill patients. Actual management issues and decision-making tasks in clinical settings for specific patient groups are seldom addressed.

In the 1990s there has been escalating public attention regarding right-to-die issues, prompted in part by the extreme position taken by Dr. Jack Kevorkian, and by legislative initiatives in several states. As noted on the front page of *The New York Times* (Scott, 1994, p. A1), "The deaths of Jacqueline Kennedy Onassis and Richard Nixon, each after rejecting medical treatment that could have prolonged their lives, appear to be accelerating the sea of change in Americans' approach to death . . . After years in which the process of dying has increasingly become the domain of doctors, *more and more Americans are trying to take back control of the time, place and circumstances of their deaths* [italics added]."

Despite the large extent of private thought on the issue of ending life for the very ill AIDS patient, there has been minimal professional exchange devoted to the subject. It is our belief that, if care providers attend to cues and events that patients respond to and become familiar with the tasks and roles they may carry out in this context, such dialogues may be facilitated.

We believe that people who are about to die have the right to determine the timing of their deaths. We also believe, based on clinical experience, that acknowledgement of this right provides a sense of personal control that often helps to sustain people and to extend the duration of their willingness to live. We emphatically do not believe or advocate that people end their lives because they have AIDS.

Any discussion of this subject must be predicated on the assumption that the patient who is considering when to die does not have significantly reduced mental capacity or clinical depression. For those who become demented in late-stage illness, and who have earlier articulated their wishes either in the form of a written health proxy or in explicit conversations with the health professional or clergy involved, we believe it acceptable to consider wishes to end life. In the absence of earlier discussions, if the patient is currently demented, we do not believe professionals are in a position to participate in such decisions unless partner, care partner, or family ask for advice and accept responsibility for any decisions that are made.

The transition from struggle to hopeless passivity and a preoccupation with ending one's misery often occurs in the context of clinical depression even in the absence of medical illness of any kind. For those who are clinically depressed and for whom death does not appear imminent, treatment for depression is indicated as a necessary step prior to consideration of the wish to die.

A word about language. We have no way of describing in neutral terms the event to which we refer: *control of the timing* of what is perceived to be inevitable and impending death by both patient and health care provider. The intent is to maintain the patient's sense of mastery and dignity on his or her terms. In this context, we do not consider the term "suicide" to be accurate. People with AIDS, instead, sometimes refer to autonomy and control. Perhaps "self-determined" or "accelerated" death are the nonjudgmental terms that come closest to describing this issue.

READINESS TO DIE

While some very sick people struggle (tenaciously, hopefully, valiantly, angrily) to the hour of death, others reach a decision at some point that "enough is enough" and that they are ready to die. There is no way to tell how often this occurs or to identify for whom or under what circumstances, since the issue is seldom discussed. The phenomenon has been observed for years, of course, but traditionally the patient is hospitalized, usually elderly, and has often became debilitated slowly over a period of years.

AIDS patients are unusual both for their youth and the often rapid progression of serious illness. Moreover, unlike other groups of patients, they are treated at home even when very ill. The greater availability of sophisticated home care and changes in insurance reimbursement policies leading to earlier discharges of sicker patients, give people with AIDS the option of dying at home. Many express this preference.

When and why do people stop actively seeking treatment, shifting to wishing to end their lives? Is there any way to predict who will do so? Some people are ready to die before medical experts consider them "end-stage," while others continue to fight under circumstances that most would consider intolerable. A care provider who is himself HIV positive observed: "When you see some of the people who are truly emaciated, you just think, would I have gone this far? And would it be so bad? Would it be so bad to be emaciated in bed? Is it worth being alive at that point? What good does it do to lie there? Why prolong it? Would there be something to gain intellectually or spiritually from this experience? It's really tough to figure out."

Pain

We asked 53 AIDS long-term survivors living at least 3 years after diagnosis of an opportunistic infection a series of questions about suicidal ideation and attempts, thoughts about living and dying, and the maintenance and diminution of hope. One question was whether there had ever been a period of a week or more "when you wanted to die." Roughly one third of the sample said "yes." We found that the circumstances surrounding a wish to die were similar: wanting to die was almost always linked to serious, debilitating illness, often entailing hospitalization, and usually accompanied by pain. For example, one man said, "I wanted to die when I had herpes over my whole body, and it smelled, and I was in terrible pain." Treatments were effective, pain was relieved, and thoughts of dying then dissipated. When feeling rested, comfortable, and alert, no man in this study reported persistent thoughts about wanting to die. When illness and pain are treatable and treated, hope is restored and life again becomes valued.

Quality of Life

It is noteworthy that one quarter of these men had made arrangements to end their lives should things become intolerable. What is striking about their statements is that many of them were living lives that those who are not ill might consider already intolerable. Nevertheless, the definition of what was "intolerable" was continually revised as limitations mounted. One man, for example, had been diagnosed with MAI (*Mycobacterium avium intracellulare* complex). An amputee prior to AIDS, his prosthesis no longer fit because of progressive weight loss. Indoors, he crawled because he was too weak for crutches; outdoors, he used a wheelchair. He lived alone and remained independent. After his AIDS diagnosis he went to graduate school at night for a masters degree, but later became too ill to work. When asked about when he would consider ending his life, he replied:

> If I get to the point where the MAI totally invades my body and where I've lost bowel function, and it progresses to my lungs. It's already gripped my liver. When I'm in too much pain and in a hopeless situation, I fantasize about going to Holland and getting a doctor to put me to sleep. I know AIDS is going to kill me, MAI actually. I know that the disease is progressing. I want quality of life, not quantity, and the quality has been damn good.

This capacity to redefine a life worth living in the face of progressive decline probably accounts for the low rates of depressive disorder we found in this long-term survivor study. As noted, these men are not representative of all people with AIDS or, for that matter, the American public in general. Some patients, lacking this outlook, may wish or choose to die before it becomes biologically necessary. This may or may not occur within the context of clinical depression.

Privacy, Dignity, and Control

Theoretical and practical questions can influence thinking about ending one's life. On a theoretical level, people with AIDS often mention three conditions they would consider unacceptable: dementia, pain, and incontinence. More abstractly, these conditions signify the loss of privacy, dignity, and control, which have emerged as defining characteristics of lives worth living in the context of AIDS. Other seriously ill patient groups have expressed similar concerns (Pearlman et al, 1993).

Practical considerations center on the quality of a person's life at home. Are there other people around besides the paid professionals? Are there visitors, companions, relatives? Can financial resources provide occasional amenities like taxis, restaurant meals, movie rentals, or attractive food for the homebound? Or, is the patient trapped in a one-room apartment crammed with medical paraphernalia and equipment, 24-hour nurses or home attendants, with no privacy, no money, no visitors, and no diversions? Such considerations are necessarily subjective, related to the person's past experiences and central values.

Friendship and Losses

Long-established friendships and even networks of acquaintances contribute immeasurably to the quality of life. A particularly wearing and insidious aspect of living with AIDS in a high-risk community is seeing friends die. As one man explained, "One by one you watch them go. The people that you lean on, that you look to for companionship, for good times, for encouragement. And the longer you live, the more losses there are. After a while it is grief beyond believing." The death of friends often results in an increased sense of personal vulnerability. "I'm very surprised at how affected I am by the deaths of my peers," one person explained. "It really felt like an insurance policy to be able to name four or five people who had AIDS longer than me. Right now, with the death of J. last week, I'm the longest surviving PWA [person with AIDS] that I know. AIDS does seem to get everybody eventually."

Not only do people with AIDS see their friends or family members dying from the same disease, but fewer and fewer people remain to turn to for comfort. In some ways it is comparable to the progressive losses of the very old who outlive their contemporaries. As their friends die, they may start to think about dying themselves and, indeed, may look forward to doing so. This is perhaps most poignant when one person with AIDS nurses a partner through the final illness. AIDS specialists have discovered that the surviving partner is at high risk for rapid decline. One physician observed, "The year after a lover loses a lover is really critical in terms of that person's survival." This also is true for the HIV-positive parent whose child dies of AIDS.

Some people can go on without friends, or they retain the health and energy to make new ones. For others, the sadness and loneliness diminish the incentive to keep going. Similar vulnerability after bereavement has been reported in studies of elderly widows (Parkes et al, 1969).

Blind and Homebound

Two significant physical events have been mentioned both by patients and physicians as landmarks in the decline of perceived quality of life and the will to live. These are AIDS-related loss of vision (usually cytomegalovirus [CMV]-induced) and the loss of mobility due to pain from neuropathy, weakness associated with wasting, or chronic and overwhelming fatigue. These events usually occur only in late-stage illness and almost always accompany or follow other major losses of physical and behavioral functioning. Blindness, together with immobility, is particularly devastating, robbing the person of both privacy and independence. Under such circumstances, while some continue to struggle tenaciously to enjoy what they can, others consider their lives no longer worth struggling for.

Turning Points and Markers

At some point people recognize that their course is running inexorably downhill. There is the growing realization of the chronicity of the illness: "I'm not going to get better. This isn't going to be intermittent anymore. It's not like before where I had episodes but then I got better." Chronic symptoms begin to wear people down, even if they are not medically serious in themselves. Persistent low-grade fever, mild nausea, pain from neuropathy, and fatigue mean that there is never a day without distress and reminders of illness.

Changes in treatment may take on special significance. Willingness to be treated with increasingly potent pain medication, for instance, may be seen to represent "surrender" to the disease. While virtually everyone agrees to take acetaminophen, and most will accept an oral opiate analgesic, some will set limits beyond that. They say, in essence, "I'm not that bad." Others are not willing to take a particular narcotic because of negative associations. One man who refused such a pain medication said, "My lover had lymphoma, and then he took MS Contin and died." The medication acquired special meaning for him as an indicator of advanced illness. Among recovering addicts, the use of opiate analgesics for pain may be avoided because they fear readdiction.

People also perceive their illness as progressing when the number of tangible reminders of illness increases. For some, AZT may become a reminder three or four times a day that something is wrong. Nevertheless, pills can be put away in a cabinet. Intravenous therapy via a central line, on the other hand, may be the constant reminder that says, "I'm sicker now and there's no reversing this." The pumps, the poles, the tubes are a physical confirmation that something is very different and worse.

Dependence on Others

One consequence of becoming chronically sicker that is particularly difficult for people who had prided themselves on their autonomy is the need to let others do things for them. In later stages of illness, friends, home aides, and nurses assume tasks and responsibilities that the patient can no longer accomplish on his or her own. Surviving at that point "often requires the ability to just sit back and accept your life being taken over by other people.

Recognizing the "End" of the Story

To understand how, why, and when people with HIV illness believe that they have come to the ends of their lives, the "story" of AIDS must be spelled out. For the general public, and even in the opinion of some members of affected communities, it is still believed that AIDS equals death. For people with AIDS and those who spend time with them, however, the "story" is far more complex, with multiple stages, steps, and events along the road.

Indeed, one of the most difficult aspects of HIV illness on a personal level is the uncertainty of what will happen next. Nevertheless, the overall shape and trajectory of the story are important in that they serve to organize both the anticipation and experience of illness.

Generally, the aggregate "story line" goes something like this:

- You get infected, but you're generally well for quite some time.
- After a while, you may begin to develop some symptoms.
- At some point, you begin medications but still go about the business of everyday life.
- Later on, you are likely to get sicker and may have to work less or not at all. More of your attention and effort become devoted to your medical care. You have more doctors' appointments, more pills, more procedures.
- After an uncertain period of time, infections may develop that require infusion therapy.
- If you have CMV, which is becoming increasingly common, you may eventually lose some or all of your vision.
- Weight loss and wasting may cause weakness and reduce mobility, and you look sick. If you get emaciated, you may need to start intravenous feeding.
- At some point, you may become largely housebound, with nurses and aides coming in.
- Eventually you are likely to be started on morphine and then you're going to die.

This story line may appear unrelievedly grim, but it is not. What is crucial to appreciate is that there is room for meaningful and potentially gratifying life at every step between diagnosis and death. Options may become restricted; changes in goals, behavior and social activities may be necessary; and horizons may become foreshortened, but the week, the day, the hour can continue to be worthwhile. The quality of hope can be preserved for nearly the entire "journey."

The story line is important because the decision to die is made when individual patients feel that they have reached the "end of the line." This need not be viewed as a form of psychopathology or a failure of hope. Sometimes the decision is accompanied by a measure of relief, since the process of dying can be more distressing than the notion of death itself. And for some, hope about survival becomes transmuted into a sense of "something" after death that they are now prepared to face.

THE ROLE OF RELIGIOUS FAITH AND SPIRITUALITY
Religious faith may play a part in decisions about ending life. It matters both for people who are sick and dying and ready to exit and for people who are not ready but who are trying to apply perspective and reason to why they are sick. Faith can clarify questions about when to stop and when and why to

keep going. Faith may make a person less ambivalent about ending his or her life. For Christians, the concepts of salvation and of eternal life may provide solace. For all people, the notions of rejoining those who already died, and, more generally, of 'something' after death, can be immensely comforting.

We recognize that no Western religion endorses active and intentional termination of one's life. However, many people with AIDS have already felt alienated from organized religion. For example, the vast majority of gay men with AIDS have already come to terms with discrepancies between the dogma of their church and their personal beliefs regarding homosexuality and have learned to set aside many of the injunctions of church leaders. Their relationship to God is often expressed personally rather than through institutional worship. Overall, we consider those who can call on some kind of religious faith to have an extra source of strength as they approach death.

Having someone to talk to about dying, or spiritual matters in general, can be extremely helpful. Not every health care provider, however, is skilled at talking about death and the hereafter. One sick patient raised the issue with his doctor, asking what he thought happened after death. The physician replied: "You go into a tunnel and you never get out of that tunnel, it's just dark." That was the physician's concept of death. It absolutely terrified the patient and made things much harder for him. A more effective intervention was related by a patient's friend:

> Last fall when Robert was sick, he entertained the idea of killing himself. For the 5 years I've known him, his spiritual faith was, "There was no God, there was no afterlife. You were dead and that's it." That was his spiritual belief. But as he got sicker, he began to think that maybe that wasn't the case. Robert became more unclear about ending his life. He began having regular conversations with a priest who would come to the hospital and to his home. After about 2 months, surrounded by his family in his hospital room, he said to the priest, "I would like to pray with my family. Will you help us pray?" The next day Robert decided to start morphine, and he died 3 days later. He came to some sort of understanding, spiritually, of what was true for him.

Clergy, especially chaplains who choose to work with AIDS patients, are usually comfortable talking about dying, and God, and the hereafter, and sometimes serve in medical settings where they are available to come to the patient's bedside. Others also can help patients sort out their thoughts, if only by listening. Although gay men and drug users are often alienated from formal religious institutions, few remain atheists as their illness progresses (just as there are said to be no atheists in foxholes). One man, diagnosed with an opportunistic infection 3 years earlier and ill for at least 6 years said, " I have very strong views, mostly negative, about organized religion, yet I consider that I have a very close relationship with God. I pray and ask for God's help and I usually use Christian imagery in my prayer. You asked me, in despair what do I do for comfort? I have turned to prayer with success."

TASKS FOR PROFESSIONAL CARE PROVIDERS

Difficult Discussions

Most of us growing up in America in the 20th century have been fortunate enough to have little direct experience with death. In our society, most people die in old age, in a hospital. As Lewis Thomas (1992) put it, "Our idea about death is that it only takes place privately, in the dark, away from other people." Furthermore, we have come to think of dying "as though it were a failure, humiliation, losing a game in which there ought to be winners." It is almost as though death is not part of life.

Health care providers are no better than others in confronting death. Indeed, physicians tend to see death as a failure of their medical science. Medical school curricula seldom address effective methods of managing death, including providing comfort for the patient and support for the family (Dubler, 1993). Even raising the issue of controlling the timing of dying has emotional, legal, and moral implications that are easier to avoid than to confront.

Most AIDS caregivers are seldom prepared by their prior professional experience to work with patients who will die. While oncologists are familiar with cancer patients who want to end their lives, AIDS specialists trained in infectious disease medicine or general medicine are accustomed to curing their patients rather than dealing with death. Similarly, psychotherapists and psychiatrists, as well as nurses who provide home care, may not be prepared for this kind of dialogue.

In a thoughtful essay concerning cancer treatment that applies to all life-threatening illnesses, Lerner (1994) observed:

> We must all face death. But the way we face it can make an extraordinary difference . . .Our culture has made dying a toxic subject. But many cultures accept death as an integral part of life. We can detoxify it by facing it, by studying the great religious and philosophical literature on death and talking about it with people we care about. Anyone who has worked with patients facing death knows that the extraordinary spiritual and psychological healing that sometimes emerges is a gift. Learning to cope with grief in life's final moments, and helping to lessen the grief of others, makes a profound difference (p 96).

Sooner or later, HIV physicians must become involved in the subject of their patients' mortality. They need to know their patients' wishes with regard to resuscitation, and withholding or terminating treatments that are no longer effective. Thus, professionals are faced with several necessary tasks when a very ill person says, "I'm ready to go." First, the professional must evaluate whether this decision is associated with clinical depression. Second, the professional must be certain that the patient has been informed about the best available medical treatment, including pain management and other palliative measures, and has received such care or has knowingly refused it. Third, while assisting the patient in thinking through the meaning of such a decision, the professional must also consider the nature of his or her own participation. Finally, the professional can help both patients and those around them to negotiate the dying process with more ease and comfort.

Talking about dying is seldom comfortable. Even when considering accelerating the process of dying, patients may need help in thinking through the timing of the decision or whether it is theirs to make at all. Preferably, such discussions begin when the person has recognized the possibility of dying but is not extremely sick. Then it may be helpful to ask: "If you get sicker, how would you want to be treated? Where do you want to be? What is your vision of the way things should be for you?" If the person seems unclear, it may helpful to tell stories about other patients to illustrate some options.

It is not uncommon among recovering substance abusers or members of the gay community to have a therapeutic relationship with a rehabilitation counselor or psychotherapist. Such a person may be the first to hear the patient's thoughts on the timing of death. As patients get sicker and mobility becomes limited, visits to counselors and therapists may end—unless the latter are flexible enough to make home and hospital visits, which is very rare. Maintenance of this therapeutic relationship can be enormously helpful as the person becomes very ill. If the patient is amenable, physicians, friends, and family members should make every effort to encourage such continued contact. (See also Chapter 12.)

Ruling Out Manageable Distress
Palliative Care. Before considering a patient's request to end life, the professional must be confident that the patient has been informed about and offered access to all available options to promote comfort and ease pain. Pain can be controlled in nearly all cases, and measures can be introduced to maximize comfort. This is not the time to be concerned about niceties, such as the potentially addictive nature of opiate analgesics, even if the person with AIDS has a history of illicit drug use. Unfortunately, the ability to provide acceptable comfort and pain control for patients at the end of life is often seen as inadequate in practice, as reflected in renewed public interest in assisted dying, as well as surveys of health professionals. (See Chapter 6 for a more detailed discussion of pain management.)

Although discomfort is usually defined in terms of pain, other conditions may cause intolerable discomfort even when pain is minimal or absent. These include severe, unremitting diarrhea, with or without incontinence; periods of mental confusion or delirium that may be direct effects of HIV or medication-induced; intractable nausea and vomiting; protracted dizziness and loss of balance; or significant loss of mobility due to muscle weakness, paralysis, neuropathy, wasting, or profound lethargy. When they are chronic, treatment-resistant, and multiple, these conditions may lead to the conclusion that life is no longer worth living.

Depression. Ideally, a professional who has known the patient over a period of time is best equipped to assess the current quality of life and whether the patient is depressed. While mental health professionals are specifically trained to identify clinical depression, they are not often involved in late-stage illness, particularly once the person with AIDS becomes homebound. Although some home-care agencies are beginning to provide mental health services to homebound clients, this is rare. Counselors who have known the person for months may be in a position to identify significant mood changes. Home-care nurses often start working with people who still can go out and enjoy activities. Consequently, they too may be able to distinguish between depression and simple physical deterioration accompanied by exhaustion. Similarly, physicians may notice gradual, or abrupt, mood changes during visits that become spaced more closely with advancing illness. Experienced clinicians usually can "rule in" depression with confidence; it is more difficult to be certain about its absence.

If a patient wishes to accelerate a death that is anticipated in 2 hours or 2 days, there is no room for therapeutic intervention other than conversation. If the time span appears to be 2 weeks or 2 months and there is some question about the presence of depression, some doctors propose a short course of stimulant medication. Effects can become apparent within 3 or 4 days, and, in some cases, there may be a dramatic difference in mood and outlook.

Even patients with histories of obvious psychiatric problems or prior suicide attempts who express a wish to die when very ill are entitled to consideration and perhaps assistance from health professionals. That is, a history of suicide attempts does not necessarily mean that the person will repeat the behavior as death approaches. A man with AIDS in his sixties who had a history of suicide attempts was remembered by a friend who was a clergyman:

> He tried to commit suicide three or four times. He had talked to me about suicide with his last diagnosis, which was terminal. And when he was first diagnosed some doctor had given him enough Seconal to kill ten people. He had never used it. And he was talking about it and talking about it. And I thought about this before I said to him, "When you're sick enough and ready to do that, I'll stay with you. You've got to be really sick enough, though, not just on a whim." And when he was at his sickest, I waited for the phone to ring. Those pills were still in the house [after he died]. He never used them.

Despite his suicide history and access to lethal medication, this man chose at the end not to take his own life. Perhaps the assurance that he had control, as well as support, sustained him.

In 1991, the Netherlands Psychiatric Association issued a policy statement on the role of psychiatrists in euthanasia, which began with this statement: "Suicide is not by definition a psychopathologic condition. The presence of psychopathology doesn't rule out the possibility of autonomous judgement in all cases... If someone with a mental illness or mental handicap requests assistance in committing suicide, the psychiatric practitioner must give due consideration to the individual's request..." (Karel, 1993). While we recognize that not all would agree, we endorse this position.

The Patient's Wishes

Advance Directives. Almost all patients with HIV illness eventually require hospitalization. Since 1991, the Federal Patient Self-Determination Act has required hospitals, nursing homes, home care agencies, and hospices "to provide patients with written information on state laws governing advance directives, and a statement of their own policies in implementing these rights" (Blendon et al, 1992). Physicians differ in their sense of timing for such discussions, although none deny their appropriateness. Some find it comfortable to bring up questions about a health proxy and living will as a routine part of intake procedures with new patients, regardless of their state of health at the time. These doctors believe it is easier to talk about such wishes when the patient is relatively healthy or at least medically stable. Others wait until there are physical indications that such discussion may be appropriate. They consider it unnecessarily upsetting to talk about issues of mortality at the beginning of a therapeutic relationship. As one physician observed, for example, "Often the first time I meet a new patient, if they're ill already, I ask if they have a power of attorney. But I worry that they think I see them as a dead person."

In 1990, a study was conducted at three health care sites in Boston to explore doctor-patient communications on resuscitation (Haas et al, 1993). Nearly 300 patients with AIDS seen either at an HMO, a public hospital clinic, or a private group practice were asked: "Have you discussed with your doctor how you wanted to be treated if your heart stops beating?" Only 38% had done so. Of the remainder, nearly three quarters wished to do so. Patients were more likely to have discussed this if they and their doctors were both white, if they had been hospitalized, if they had been diagnosed for longer than 1 year, and if they were seen in the private practice setting. Length of doctor-patient relationship and characteristics of the physician other than race were not associated with discussion of preferences. These results suggest that the large majority of patients do wish to talk to their doctors about issues related to dying, although half of those who want to, don't.

Health Proxy. It is expected that such conversations include the patient's designation of a "health proxy," a person who is authorized to make health care decisions ranging from hospital admission or discharge to decisions about life-sustaining procedures. The more explicit the written health care proxy and medical directive, the more effective it is. Gay Mens' Health Crisis Inc. has prepared a detailed sample directive (see Appendix III) that enumerates multiple options that the patient either requests or refuses to accept under specific circumstances, such as permanent coma or substantial and irreversible loss of mental functions. Choice of a health proxy warrants considerable thought. One's partner, mother, or best friend may not be the most prudent choice, since they may be unwilling to set aside their own passionate convictions about survival to honor the patient's wishes. A neutral person may be more effective as a proxy.

A medical directive is useful only if it is available to medical or hospital staff at the time decisions must be made. Copies should be given to the appointed proxy and also kept in hospital charts as well as with the physician's medical records. Otherwise, those present when a crisis occurs may not be aware of the existence of the directive or the identity of the proxy who should be contacted.

Decisions about terminating treatment or withholding life-sustaining equipment usually do not, and should not present legal or ethical dilemmas for health care providers, assuming the patient's wishes are known. Decision-making can become far more complicated and ambiguous when the patient is not actively dying or when medical directives do not apply. The care provider may be faced with an ambulatory patient who asks for a barbiturate prescription because of chronic but not immediately life-threatening distress (such as treatment-resistant low-grade pain, fever, and fatigue). Or, a bedridden patient, already receiving I.V. morphine, with weeks more to live may ask the physician to hasten an inevitable but not immediately impending death.

A particularly poignant example of the complexity and difficulty of these decisions is the patient with cognitive involvement who fears he or she will be incompetent to make such decisions in the foreseeable future. As a dying patient featured in the cover story of a *New York Times Magazine* article said, "I'm tired. I'm in constant pain. I'm getting weaker by the day. I want to do this at home, before my body's here and my brain isn't" (Belkin, 1993). When health care providers are asked for help in access to the means of death (writing prescriptions or nursing orders), this is a request for assisted suicide.

Hospice Care. In theory, hospice care fulfills many of the requirements of doctors and patients. In fact, according to a 1992 Gallup poll, nine of ten Americans prefer this option (Cerquone, 1992). Hospice teams help families to manage the patient at home, are constantly available for support, and provide optimal palliative care. However, the underlying assumptions of hospice are that death is expected within 6 months, and that aggressive medical care, which is no longer useful, will not be provided. For patients with AIDS, the point at which these assumptions may be made may be unclear. Nevertheless, if this option is geographically available, it warrants discussion.

Euthanasia and HIV. Direct aid in dying is both legally and ethically complicated. It is, however, an age-old dilemma. The Hippocratic oath would not have addressed the question unless ancient physicians had been asked, and the oath specifies: "I will give no deadly drug to any patient though it be asked of me." This is regarded by some physicians as an absolute prohibition. Other components of the Hippocratic Oath have, however, been universally discarded without controversy (such as the mandate to "look upon him who has taught me this Art even as one of my parents...[and] teach [his offspring] this Art, if they would learn it, without fee or covenant." Consequently, a fundamentalist approach to the Hippocratic Oath, like one to the Bible, must address the selective nature of the rules that are considered immutable.

Although no physician has so far been convicted of "mercy killing" in an American court, it is illegal to actively assist a suicide. It is not, however, illegal to be present. On the other hand, it is considered both legal and ethical in traditional medical ethics and by many religious groups to prescribe and provide treatment intended to relieve suffering, even if the "unintended" additional effect of such treatment is to hasten death. A handbook of pain management for the terminally ill patient, published by the Washington State Medical Society (1992) notes, "It is professionally and ethically correct to increase the dose of medication even to the point of risking death provided the primary goal of the physician is to alleviate pain." This is referred to as the doctrine of double effect. It is in this context that the dose of morphine may be increased to alleviate pain even though it eventually will slow respiration to the point where life cannot be sustained.

There are at least two fairly distinct phases of illness when HIV physicians may be asked for assistance in dying. A substantial number of HIV patients seek, in advance, to have "the means" available to them, should they get sick enough to consider their lives intolerable (Rabkin et al, 1993). This usually means a request for assisted suicide, such as a prescription for barbiturates as recommended by Humphrey in his book *Final Exit* (1992). When this request is made, the patient is typically medically stable and not necessarily acutely ill. The second broad category of requests arise when the patient is indeed actively dying, and this is presumably the final illness from which recovery is not expected. In this context, more active assistance by the physician is usually involved, most often by raising the dose of I.V. morphine, perhaps with the addition of diazepam or potassium chloride, which he/she may administer in person. The former is considered "assisted suicide," and the latter, euthanasia.

The Assisted Death. Physician-assisted suicide for AIDS patients still lacks a consensus within the AIDS community. Because of the varied religious, moral, legal, and ethical identities of the parties affected, different viewpoints must respectfully coexist. If doctors and patients have fundamentally different views, the patient should find a physician who shares his or her thinking.

Although few of the physicians we asked had moral reservations about assistance in dying for their patients who were very ill, some had more difficulty than others in the level of intervention they were comfortable with. The least difficult decision for a physician appears to be increasing the dose of I.V. morphine for a patient already on it:

> I think if people don't want to go on, they have the right to end things.
> What I have done, and what I do routinely is morphine. I had a very sick
> patient who was at home, and his lover, who was also a patient of mine,
> had died the week before. He said, "I'm ready for this to be over. I want to
> die. I want to be with F." Of course, he had morphine already. I said, "Look.
> This is what you do. You see that pump over there? Just keep hitting that
> pump. And have friends increase the dose. I will tell the home care com-
> pany you can titrate the dose. And I will give you valium for anxiety, and
> you ask for that valium. And I'll tell your friends to give you that valium
> if they see any muscle twitching or anything remotely indicative of dis-
> comfort." That's the quick way to do it. He died the next morning.

This doctor estimated such situations occur a couple of times a month.

Once I.V. morphine is started, some people wish to be kept comfortable
but don't want the course to be aggressive, while others want to die quickly. In the hospital, access to morphine is often available, but its titration may
be problematic. Physicians usually agree to start I.V. morphine when a
patient is clearly terminal, and orders often are written for increasing
amounts "for the control of pain." When patients become lethargic as they
are dying, or become comatose, they no longer communicate distress.
Although the intent of increasing the dose of morphine is to alleviate
pain, at sufficient doses (that vary from person to person) there is the secondary effect of slowing respiration enough to end life.

Hospital staff can become very upset about increasing morphine in such
situations. Often the physician is willing to take the chance of this "double
effect," but the nurse objects. This can lead to complaints by the nurse to the
house staff and calls to the nursing supervisor. The burden of the complaint
is that the patient is not in "subjective distress," and that morphine increases are thus not indicated. What then ensues is an explicit discussion of this
situation which, in an institutional setting, becomes difficult to manage no
matter what the health proxy says. Physicians at this point will probably
decline to increase morphine doses for the patient who is no longer communicative unless he is actually heard by the nurse to be groaning. Given the
possibility of fluctuations in level of consciousness during this period, 24-hour
surveillance would be needed to detect manifestations of distress sufficient
to meet the requirement of "documented distress." This, of course, is not provided by hospital staff. This kind of situation can occur, even though the
patient had earlier stated that he was still in pain, had explicitly stated his
wishes about accepting or advocating the second effect of higher doses of
morphine, and had the health proxy present to articulate these wishes.
Then, the patient may linger for days while the loved ones and family
wait helplessly in a death watch that the patient had made every effort to
prevent.

One physician refuses to use morphine anymore, after a disastrous experience with a patient who, despite raising his morphine to 300 mg an hour,

induced only 2 or 3 days of hallucinations and incontinence, after which he recovered. Instead, he is willing to assist in other ways when he is confident that the patient has reached a calm, clear-headed decision made over a period of time rather than an impulsive, desperate request.

This theme is widely expressed. "People who are serious about getting the means to end life need to talk to me about it over a period of time, and I need to make sure they're not temporarily depressed. And, they need to initiate the conversation. They need to do their research, bring it up again next month and the month after and then we'll see. It's a long process."

From a practical standpoint, few physicians would write a prescription for barbiturates in sufficient quantity to provide a lethal dose. Instead they will write a prescription every 10 to 20 days until a sufficient quantity has been accumulated. A single prescription for 50 tablets, for example, is uncommon and likely to be suspect, especially if the patient dies shortly thereafter.

One doctor observed:

> Assisted suicide is like abortion; very ethically minded people disagree violently about it. My feeling is that my job as a doctor is to meet the real needs and wishes of my patients. My obligation at the minimum is not to interfere, and then to help to whatever extent I feel comfortable. For some reason, and it doesn't make sense intellectually, I feel comfortable giving people pills. I don't feel comfortable going over to their house and giving them an amp of potassium. Maybe one day I will. And I also make sure that if someone is doing that, they let me know. I want to verify that they're thinking about this in a level-headed way. I give scripts [prescriptions] to a lot of people who never used them. I think it was their control button.

This physician believes that, from a technical point of view, morphine doesn't work very well. Taking a barbiturate overdose is more effective. "The problem is, a lot of people who are real sick can't keep that stuff down. If you really were using I.V.s, an amp of potassium makes plenty of sense, along with diazepam so there aren't any muscle problems. Morphine takes a long time; potassium is quick. On the other hand, you can justify morphine medically." Another physician, who acknowledged that she would use potassium if she were to kill herself, said that neither she nor other doctors she knew used it for patients because of the lack of medical justification.

These HIV specialists all had worked out conditions in which they were comfortable helping their patients to die. All had in fact done so. Further, they believed that their attitudes and behavior were common among their peers though infrequently discussed openly. One doctor in San Francisco went so far as to speculate that assistance in dying was provided by "a lot of physicians. As a matter of fact, comfort care is sort of a euphemism for euthanasia. But it isn't discussed openly, except between doctors caring for the same patient."

In 1989, a survey was conducted in San Francisco among 69 physicians belonging to an organization for HIV care providers and 86 physicians randomly selected from the state medical association's mailing list. Over half expressed no moral reluctance about providing medications for an AIDS patient who requests them in order to end life, and 24% said they would actually do so when initially asked (Slome et al, 1992). HIV specialists did not differ from the community sample of physicians in their responses.

Access and options. We strongly endorse the position that assistance in dying in the form of drug prescriptions should be provided only within the context of an ongoing therapeutic relationship, not for a patient seen once. This policy does, however, restrict assistance in dying to patients who have an established relationship with a doctor. Some people, particularly poorer people, do not have an ongoing relationship with one physician, either because they attend a clinic with rotating coverage or because they do not regularly use the same health care facility. Are they to be denied this option? Intravenous drug users and former users generally have the knowledge and access to end their own lives without assistance, but what of others?

Permission to Die. PWAs as a group show extraordinary determination, struggle for months and years with multiple changing, unpredictable medical exigencies and are oriented toward survival, not dying. The decision to die is not made lightly even when someone is clearly very ill.

Sometimes requests for permission to die are oblique. One man said to a friend (rather than his lover who had always fiercely encouraged him to keep going): "I don't think I can keep doing this too much longer. It's just too hard now." Another man expressed similar feelings: "I don't know how much longer I can go on. I'm getting weaker. Is there something to do next? Should I do something, or just let it happen?" Although there is clearly no right answer, it is our general belief that our role is not to give permission for one choice or another, but to affirm the person's right to make his or her own decision. After listening and perhaps asking questions, we might eventually say, "It's up to you and your God. It's your life and your choice. There's a limit to how much anyone can take, but only you can decide when that limit is reached."

Judgments about the nature of virtue and courage sometimes complicate these considerations. Most of us have been raised to believe, at least to some extent, that it is noble to endure, harking back to Augustine's fifth century view that "life and its suffering were divinely ordained by God and must be borne accordingly" (Hamel, 1991). People who are healthy tend to define courage in a terminal illness as "fighting to the last." The decision to end life "prematurely" by people with AIDS, before they are actively dying, is somehow less morally impressive. In talking to those who are themselves ill, especially those who have seen and perhaps attended to the last illness of other people with AIDS, a reversal sometimes occurs. Hearing of someone who chose to end his life, another PWA may say, "I wish I had his courage." One man said, "I refuse to struggle for my final days like a drowning rat in a pail of water. Then I will refuse to live." And he did act on this decision, which we consider also an honorable and courageous choice.

These are general considerations. Some people are prepared to struggle much longer than others. Each person has different trajectories or objectives that sustain them. Some people simply get tired, even in the absence of identifiable changes. "I am being worn down by this. It does not get easier. It gets harder. I worry that I'll reach a point where I'll give up and won't be able to endure what I go through, although I do my best to resist such feelings." Another put it this way: "The paradox of being a long-term survivor is that it's also sometimes like long-term torture. Dying slowly really upsets me. I would sooner be taken out in the back and shot. I think that is a reason why a lot of people can't stand this anymore. You just get really tired." So one never can predict with certainty when or if someone is going to say "enough is enough."

It is far easier to believe in the right to choose the timing of one's death when the person is actively dying, when their remaining time is likely to be hours or days. The strength of this conviction is tested when the person is not acutely and severely ill and untreatable and may have weeks or months to go before an inevitable death. Such a person may be able to survive physically but with such chronic discomfort and restricted horizons that he or she sees no reason to remain alive. Is this person entitled to say, "enough is enough?" We do believe so.

Helping Make Choices. Once a person communicates, either obliquely or directly, that they want to end life, doctors and home care nurses can convey their willingness to help make choices. This includes wishes to discontinue medicine and medical procedures, deciding where they want to be when they get sicker—in the hospital or at home—and whom to have present. It also may include the more complicated question of providing the means.

Caregiving professionals, as well as relatives, may find it increasingly stressful to watch their patient or loved one decline. Those who work professionally with PWAs see them regularly and frequently over time, often have much in common with them, and may identify with the patient, their lovers, or their children. They may be willing to say, "Start the morphine," because it is their own pain and suffering that they want to deal with.

The opposite agenda may also be at work. Lovers or friends may say to an exhausted and very ill patient, "You can't give up. I need you here." Or (as was said to a poster boy AIDS activist): "You can't die. You'll be letting so many people down!" In either instance, a political or personal agenda should not be given precedence over the patient's rights and needs.

When the professional care provider learns that a patient is ready to die, and clinical depression or inadequate pain control do not appear to be the reasons, the patient's wishes should be clarified. The caregiving professional can let it be known that he or she is willing to help make choices. Patients should be encouraged to talk to those close to them while they think this through. In the unusual case that the patient decides to take action, it is essential that the health proxy and physician are informed of intent to end life: Barbiturate overdose is treatable and does not fall under the provisions of DNR orders.

As patients approach death, the obligation of health care providers should be extended not only to the patient but also to those who love him or her. One physician said as much: "When you're caring for someone who is very sick, you're really caring for all the people that love them. And they want their family to be as comfortable as possible. In the very last hours of life the patient may be breathing agonally. I don't know if that's uncomfortable for the patient, but it's very uncomfortable for their loved ones. So upping the morphine dose at that point to ensure comfort is fine, even if that means an earlier death."

Within this framework, the health care provider and even the patient may worry about the impact on loved ones of these discussions about discontinuing treatments or choosing to die. One doctor noted: "Someone's assisted suicide affects not just the doctor and the patient. In my experience the people intimately involved suffer profoundly, even though they're part of the process."

While it *is* painful to be intimately involved in the planning and witnessing of the act, in our experience it may be even more painful to be excluded. It can, in reality, be helpful for close loved ones to be intimately involved in the process. There is also pain in *not* having had a chance to say goodbye, or to know that the person died alone. Death costs, and the issue is that of relative suffering, not its presence or absence. When someone who is loved dies, there will be grief; there need not be anguish.

REFERENCES

Aries P. *The Hour of Our Death*. New York: Knopf; 1981.

Belkin L. There's no simple suicide. *New York Times Magazine*. 1993; November 14: 48ff.

Blendon R, Szalay U, Knox R. Should physicians aid their patients in Dying? A public perspective. *Journal of the American Medical Association*. 1992;267,2658-2662.

Brody H. Assisted death—a compassionate response to a medical failure. *New England Journal of Medicine*. 1992;327:1384-1388.

Cerquone J. Poll says hospice leads. *Hospice Magazine*. 1992;3:4-5.

Dubler N. Commentary: balancing life and death—proceed with caution. *American Journal of Public Health*. 1993;83:23-25.

Dworkin, R. The right to death. *The New York Review of Books*. 1991;January 31:14-17.

Haas J, Weissman J, Cleary P, et al. Discussion of preferences for life-sustaining care by persons with AIDS: predictors of failure in patient-physician communications. *Archives of Internal Medicine*. 1993;153:1241-1248.

Hamel R. *Choosing Death*. Philadelphia: Trinity Press International; 1991.

Hamel R (ed). *Choosing death: Active Euthanasia, Religion and the Public*

Debate. Philadelphia: Trinity Press International; 1991.Wolf SM. Nancy Beth Cruzan: in no voice at all. *Hastings Center Report*. 1990;20:38-41.

Hastings Center. Dying well? A colloquy on euthanasia and assisted suicide (special issue). *Hastings Center Report*. 1992;22:6-55.

Humphry D. *Final Exit: The Practicalities of Self-Deliverance and Assisted Suicide for the Dying*. New York: Dell Publishing; 1991.

Karel R. Controversy over assisted suicide cases highlights ethical issues, clinical concerns. *Psychiatric News*, 1993; December 17: 4.

Lerner M, Hedging the bet against cancer. *The New York Times Magazine*, Oct., 2, 1994, pp.64ff.

Madan TN. Dying with dignity. *Social Science & Medicine*. 1992;35:425-433.

Misbin R. Physicians' aid in dying. *New England Journal of Medicine*. 1991:325:1307-1310.

Parkes CM, Benjamin B, Fitzgerald R. Broken heart: a statistical study of increased mortality among widowers. *British Medical Journal*. 1969;1:740-743.

Pearlman R, Cain K, Patrick D, et al. Insights pertaining to patient assessments of states worse than death. *The Journal of Clinical Ethics*. 1993;4:33-41.

Quill TE, Cassel CK, Meier D. Care of the hopelessly ill: proposed clinical criteria for physician-assisted suicide. *New England Journal of Medicine*. 1992;327:1380-1384.

Rabkin JG, Remien RH, Katoff LS, et al. Resilience in adversity among longterm survivors of AIDS. *Hospital & Community Psychiatry*. 1993;44:162-167.

Scott J. An Onassis legacy: facing death on one's own terms. *The New York Times*. 1994;June 4:1A.

Slome L, Moulton J, Huffine C, et al. Physicians' attitudes toward assisted suicide in AIDS. *Journal of Acquired Immune Deficiency Syndromes*. 1992;5:712-718.

Thomas L. *The Fragile Species*. New York: Scribner's; 1992.

Wanzer SH, et al. The physician's responsibility toward hopelessly ill patients: a second look. *New England Journal of Medicine*. 1989;320:844-849.

Washington State Medical Association. *Pain Management and Care of the Terminal Patient*. Seattle, Wash: Washington State Medical Association; 1992.

Wolf SM. Nancy Beth Cruzan: in no voice at all. *Hastings Center Report*. 1990;20:38-41

12

THE ROLE OF THE COUNSELOR

COMMENT

Due to the chronic nature of the disease, as well as the youth of many of the patients, HIV requires that counselors—regardless of training—define their functions somewhat more broadly than they would in a conventional therapist-client relationship. Acute illnesses and disabilities may require, for example, that the counselor go to the patient, rather than vice versa. And very young patients may suffer from existential dilemmas generally not encountered in adults before the sixth or seventh decades. Families, friends, and the ever-present threat of death often complicate the therapist-client relationship in ways that counselors dealing with other populations do not often face. Despite the challenges of working with HIV-positive and AIDS clients, however, the rewards of helping people negotiate one of the most complex diseases humankind has ever seen can be enormous and gratifying.

THE HIV COUNSELOR: DEFINITIONS

In the evolution of HIV care, many types of professionals and lay persons have involved themselves in the task of counseling people living with HIV and AIDS. Thus, the term "counselor" must be broadly defined. The involvement of lay counselors came about, at least in part, as a result of the relatively "slow" response of professional groups in the early part of the epidemic. To fill what was perceived as a gap in needed services, "peer" counselors emerged to provide support to people coping with AIDS. Today, counselors who work with HIV and AIDS clients have had varying degrees of training as mental health providers, and they include social workers, psychologists, psychiatrists, nurses, clergy, and lay peer counselors. Counseling services can range from advice about access to health care and legal services to traditional forms of psychiatric treatment, including medical treatment of clinical depression. This chapter focuses on counseling for the problems of living with HIV illness, not on specific mental disorders.

While a comprehensive review of HIV and AIDS counseling is not possible within the scope of this book, this chapter is included to demonstrate some of the key roles that a "counselor" can play in the lives of people living with HIV and AIDS, as well as the rewards of such work. Patients, too, will be reminded of the benefits of working with someone outside of their family or friendship networks as they cope with the many challenges in their lives. [For a more comprehensive coverage of counseling issues see Caldwell et al, 1994; Winiarski, 1991; Green and McCreaner, 1989.]

A Willingness to Be Flexible

Counselors and therapists who work with HIV patients usually find that they need to be more flexible because of the nature of the disease than they are with other patients. The nature of the therapeutic relationship requires close follow-up, including home and hospital visits, in times of acute serious illness. Therapists may have different policies, for instance, about whether or not they will visit patients, make phone calls, or charge for appointments canceled at the last minute because of sudden illness. HIV counselors need to be clear with themselves and their clients about their boundaries and limits.

Even when patients are not fully conscious or able to communicate, important psychological work can continue. By his or her mere presence, as well as consistent ongoing contact, the counselor provides considerable support.

As in other chronic disease situations, counselors are likely to meet the client's significant others, providing the opportunity to assess the quality of these relationships and to offer support. It may be necessary, in fact, to redefine the "client" to include those people close to him or her, that is, the "family."

Maintaining Boundaries

Although counselors should be willing to be flexible, to be effective they must also learn to maintain boundaries. All counselors have limits in terms of what can be adequately accomplished and need to recognize that they cannot "do it all" for their clients. Many counselors, especially early in their professional lives, readily develop "magical thinking," believing that if their client does all the "right" things, perhaps he or she will never get sick. The existence of many long-term survivors and "HIV-positive non-progressors" is seductive, contributing to the belief that clients will survive. Unfortunately, counselors who feel this way are devastated when they first witness serious illness progression and/or death in one of their clients. They may even blame themselves, as clients often do, for not doing enough.

While the counselor has a specific role in the lives of his or her clients, he or she should be careful about taking on too much. The counselor cannot be confidante, family member, case manager, buddy, medical expert, best friend, and therapist all at once. Neither can the counselor be available at all times to all clients.

The importance of maintaining boundaries was illustrated by a counselor who was having difficulty coping with her client's end-stage illness. She was visiting the hospital regularly to work with her client who was grappling with the dying process. Although this was valuable time for them, the counselor became more and more involved, albeit informally, with her client's children. The children began to treat the counselor like an aunt and after some time, began to telephone her at home. The counselor began to feel overwhelmed, despairing about her work with her client. For her part, the client also had some negative feelings about the attachment she observed between the children and her counselor. A supervisor helped this counselor realize that her feelings of distress did not stem from her work with her client but resulted from a lack of clarity about the boundaries of her role and the inappropriate demands of the children. Moreover, since the relationship between the counselor and the children had never been defined or discussed, the client, understandably, had ambivalent feelings. In fact, because these issues had not been addressed, the counselor's well-intentioned interactions with the children became a barrier to effective therapy with her client. When she became aware of these issues, the counselor was able to discuss the children's needs with her client. A family therapist was asked to work with the children, allowing the counselor to continue to work closely and effectively with her client until death.

Another therapist, who for many years had worked with clients individually, found that his policy on hospital visits required modification when he began facilitating AIDS support groups. The first time a member of a group was hospitalized, the therapist went to the hospital to visit, which had always been his policy with individual clients. Shortly thereafter, however, two other members of the group became ill suddenly and were hospitalized. The therapist was not able to visit them that week. At the next group session, other members asked the facilitator about the members who were missing and wanted to know how they were doing. One group member wanted to know why he had visited John, but not Carlos or Greg. This counselor learned that he needed to establish a policy of not visiting group members in the hospital because he would not always be able to follow through. He also needed to talk about this policy explicitly with the group and to discuss what their expectations and wishes were of each other should any of them become ill. Consequently, they were able to establish a chain of communication among themselves to handle news about members who were ill and had missed group sessions.

HELPING CLIENTS NEGOTIATE THE SYSTEM

The counselor is often able to help HIV-infected clients negotiate attitudinal obstacles to care, as well as helping them to contain anger that might alienate health care providers who are willing to serve them. Clients may need information and assistance in contacting service agencies for transportation, housing, financial aid, food delivery, home health care, and domestic chores. In some areas, good case management is offered by hospital social workers or staff of community-based AIDS service organizations. In others, the counselor may be the only one able to serve in this capacity.

Sometimes people with HIV infection feel that they have to "settle for whatever they can get," believing that better or more aggressive treatment is unavailable to them because of cost, geography, or fear of discrimination. Others are plagued by numerous questions and the need to make important decisions: Should my present treatment regimen be abandoned in favor of a new one? Should I trust my physician (or clinic) or should I switch to a different one?" These questions often lead to ruminative anxiety which can make it extremely difficult for the HIV-infected person to get on with his or her life. Since the therapist can play a crucial role in helping patients sort out these emotionally charged issues, counselors need to be well informed about treatment of HIV and AIDS. While they will not be making decisions for their patients, they still need to be familiar with the context and issues that their clients are confronting.

Working with HIV-infected clients requires counselors to become involved in the community, regardless of where the community is located, to find out what is offered and where and to build working relationships with key providers at agencies that offer assistance to people with HIV infection. People with AIDS often need support, guidance, and concrete information when making decisions about ceasing to work, obtaining Social Security benefits, accessing drug treatment programs, and arranging for psychosocial support services. Accurate and knowledgeable guidance by a counselor can be invaluable to restoring the client's sense of independence and control.

PSYCHOLOGICAL ISSUES

Accelerated Adult Development

Erik Erikson is probably most well known for his theory that people continue to develop beyond childhood, that there are discrete stages of adult development, and that individuals are propelled from one stage to the next by crises (Erikson, 1959). And, Carl Jung described the second half of adult life as an opportunity for new directions and new challenges in interpersonal relationships, as well as for a new and deeper relationship with one's own inner life (Jung, 1960).

When people encounter HIV disease in the middle of this developmental process—at age 30 or 40, or even younger—their vistas suddenly shrink. The endpoint of life is perceived as moving closer. A decline in health status may hasten the psychological process of aging, which may, in turn, accelerate adult development. According to Erikson's model, in the final stage of development, people either achieve "ego integrity" (a feeling of completeness and satisfaction with life's accomplishments) or fall into a state of despair. Thomas (1994) found that a sample of gay men (HIV-positive and HIV-negative) living in New York City and a geriatric sample, were at a similar stage of adult development even though the mean age of the gay cohort was 41.

Certain crises and challenges typically confront people at specific stages of HIV infection. At such times, the counselor can provide crisis management, support, and stability, and thus facilitate growth and development.

Providing a Safe Place to Express Intense Emotions

People living with HIV and AIDS experience a wide range of emotional reactions to the actual, as well as the anticipated, events in their lives. They may feel hopeful, calm, and connected one day, and pessimistic, fearful and alienated on another. When counselors validate this wide range of feelings as normal, the patient can typically "ride the roller coaster" without undue panic and without "falling apart." Counselors can also provide a safe environment in which the patient can express any and all feelings. This can be particularly important, since patients may be reluctant to express all of their feelings with lovers, spouses, close friends, family members, or acquaintances. This is often at least partly out of a desire to "protect" or "spare" loved ones the burden of profound fears and often intense emotions. Further, patients may not want to share their fears with their primary health care provider, for example, in order to preserve the focus of that relationship on the medical management of their disease.

Benefits and Risks of Denial

A certain degree of denial can be useful for people living with HIV. Since the course of HIV illness is unpredictable for most people, it is important to be able to accept the notion of a long-term future with good health and things to look forward to. One might even consider the possibility of extended survival where eventual death is caused by some unrelated illness, much later in life. Some would call this denial—others call it maintaining hope.

Denial is selfish and risky, however, when it interferes with the need to protect a sexual partner or with the need to act on real symptoms and acute medical events. The importance of honesty between patient and health care provider is essential in promoting aggressive and timely medical management of this disease. Counselors can address the issue of denial in a supportive manner: They can talk about the normal desire to "forget" or "just not think about it for awhile," while pushing clients to confront the realities of this disease in very concrete and practical terms. Taking mental "HIV vacations" can provide a welcome respite, as long as the real demands of health care management are not altogether denied.

Disclosure of HIV Status

The subject of disclosure typically arises at some point in most counseling situations. Counselors can and should encourage candor between clients and their sex- and needle-sharing partners and should discuss issues of safer and less safe behaviors in a non-judgmental manner. It is also important that counselors acknowledge the difficulty in both initiating and maintaining certain behavioral changes. Discussions about disclosure of HIV status to others are useful and appropriate, since this can be an emotionally charged topic. Therapists can help patients resist both the desire to withdraw and isolate themselves, refusing to tell anyone, or the opposite, to "tell the world." Neither extreme response is adaptive. The counseling situation is an excellent place to discuss the pros and cons of disclosure to certain people;

whom to tell first, second, etc.; the best way to tell (i.e., in person, in a letter, by telephone); and the optimal time to tell. Role playing can be a useful technique to help facilitate the disclosure process as well as ease the client's anxieties.

The following case is presented to illustrate how the counselor can play a key role in helping clients process decisions associated with disclosure, which can cause anxiety, confusion, and even emotional paralysis. Although there is no right way to disclose painful truths to loved ones, here is an example of how one individual and his therapist tackled the problem.

CASE #1: Ben

Ben was a 34-year-old gay man living in New York City. He had a large family including an 83-year-old mother, three brothers, three sisters, and several nieces and nephews that lived in different parts of the country. Ben was ambivalent about telling his family about his HIV diagnosis. He wondered whether it was right to cause his mom to "worry about him at her age?" In fact, why should any of them worry about him? What could they do about it anyway? And, he was still healthy. Most of his family didn't even know he was gay. Would it be too much to come out about being gay and being HIV-positive?

After discussing this and several related issues in counseling over a few months, Ben realized that he wanted his family to know because he wanted the support from them—if it were there to be had. Also, he wanted them to know about his HIV status while he was healthy rather than waiting until he was sick.

With his counselor, Ben explored his options and discussed the pros and cons of each. Role playing his "worst case scenario" let him see that it probably would not be as bad as he feared and significantly reduced his anxiety.

After much discussion, Ben decided, with his counselor, to first inform those he felt closest to and to listen to their advice about informing the rest of the family. After doing this, he wrote to the other siblings, informing them of the news and then spoke with them by telephone. All, except one, called Ben shortly after receiving the news and offered their love and support.

As a group, they decided that their mother should be told, that she had great inner strength and deserved to be included. They planned a family reunion so that they would all be together over several days. Ben was able to tell her, and the family had several days afterwards to deal with their feelings and express support for Ben.

The Blues Versus Depression: What Is Normal?

Although early reports indicated high degrees of psychopathology in gay men infected with HIV (Dilley et al, 1985; Nichols, 1985; Tross et al, 1987; Atkinson et al, 1988), more recent studies have found no significant differences in rates of psychiatric distress and depressed mood compared with

HIV-seronegative controls (Satz et al, 1988; Ostrow et al, 1989) or community samples matched by gender and age (Williams et al, 1991). In fact, a comprehensive review of published research on the prevalence of psychiatric disorders across diverse populations with HIV disease found no consistent pattern of psychiatric diagnoses nor a typical diagnosis (Bialer et al, 1991).

A recent study of male AIDS long-term survivors reported that in spite of multiple illnesses, stressors, losses, and a wide range of physical impairments, these men exhibited low aggregate rates of syndromal mood disorders and psychiatric distress (Rabkin et al, 1993). When present, symptoms of depression and anxiety were mild and unrelated to degree of physical impairment. While transient distress is common, clinical depression is not the norm for many people living with HIV. Structured forms of psychotherapy or pharmacology have been effective in relieving depression, even in patients with severe immune suppression (Markowitz, Rabkin, and Perry, 1994; Rabkin et al, 1994). Since some of the symptoms of depression, such as lethargy and sleep or appetite disturbances, also can be caused by HIV illness, counselors without diagnostic expertise are advised to refer clients to experts in this area.

Substance Abuse

Many people living with HIV and AIDS also have problems with persistent or periodic substance abuse. This cannot be ignored nor denied. Such behaviors must be addressed with the client and considered in the overall management plan. Although most experts in the field advise incorporating substance abuse treatment into other HIV-related services, this is an ideal situation that is only sometimes achieved in the real world. Counselors who work with HIV-infected people need to be sensitive to the need for substance abuse treatment, and to realize that provision of such services requires special training. Referral to or consultation with experts is recommended (Mulleady, 1992).

Suicide

As with clinical depression, there have been some reports of elevated risk for suicidal thinking, suicide attempts, and suicide in people with AIDS (Marzuk et al, 1988; Frierson and Lippmann, 1988; Kizer, et al., 1988). In their review, Beckett et al (1993) found factors such as social support, meaningful work, and religious beliefs key to diminishing the chance of suicide. They also observed that HIV-seropositive people without AIDS are more likely to exhibit suicidal ideation than those with AIDS. In the study of AIDS long-term survivors, no suicide attempts were made by anyone except those with a previous history of such attempts. None reported current suicidal ideation, although several considered it a future option should their condition become intolerable (Rabkin et al, 1993).

The therapist is obliged to assess suicidality and respond to it as he or she would with any other client. Therefore a diagnosis of clinical depression must be considered, together with a thorough assessment of physical pain.

Counselors also need to be able to distinguish between acute suicidality, which is rare, and a kind of contingency plan—killing oneself if certain medical developments such as blindness, paralysis, disfigurement, or chronic pain were to occur. Although many patients believe that they might choose suicide at some future point, when severe physical problems do develop, they often discover new strengths and renegotiate the circumstances in which they would end their lives.

Therapists should make it clear that choosing the time of one's death is a legitimate option, as well as a topic always open for discussion. Serious consideration of how and when one might choose to die ultimately returns to clients a sense of control and reduces affective distress. Knowing that death is in one's own hands can restore emotional equilibrium and the energy and motivation to engage in life again.

The Meaning of Life

For some individuals, a positive HIV test result or a diagnosis of AIDS signifies the prospect of impending death, with the sense that there is no time left. For others, the concept of a disease that may kill them in several years poses relatively little threat compared to the daily risks of staying alive on the street. For many, however, confronting the possibility of death due to HIV leads to serious consideration of existential questions: What is the purpose of my life and how do I derive meaning from the time I have left? An individual's identity may undergo significant change as he or she tries to redefine the self within the context of a perceptually more limited time frame. Clients normally pass through all the stages of grief as they mourn the loss of the self that they used to be. Adjusting to seropositive status is a process of integrating new information about oneself into one's existing identity. This process necessarily includes questioning assumptions about one's life, redefining priorities, establishing new goals, and acquiring new skills. It is an effort that takes time and can also evoke a sequence of grief, loss, and rage in many people. This journey often becomes the focus of therapy with HIV-positive clients.

TRANSITIONS

There are specific times in the course of HIV disease during which patients are particularly vulnerable to acute distress, such as at first confirmation of positive HIV status; at the initial onset of physical symptoms; during a sudden decline in CD4+ cells; or during the first opportunistic infection. Continuing to maintain hope in the face of illness progression, despite grim predictions about the chance for a "cure," is a considerable psychological challenge for patients and care providers. Hope is extremely important throughout the process of HIV infection, but especially during acute illness when it is more likely to be undermined.

For clients who had been asymptomatic, the emergence of symptoms can be terrifying, symbolizing the progression of the disease or the beginning of the end. Panic reactions are common. Because physical symptoms may signify failure, especially in clients who have been particularly successful at taking charge of their own health, the onset of new symptoms can produce feelings of depression, self-reproach, and guilt. For many, hospitalization is the turning point, underscoring the transformation from "asymptomatic" to having AIDS.

For some, the second opportunistic infection is truly devastating. There may be a complete recovery, for instance, after a first illness, with a return to a "normal" life. Getting sick again, however, is a very real reminder that "it's not over" and will probably get worse. To minimize the distress, some clients minimize the significance of new symptoms and avoid treatment, while others deny the presence of symptoms altogether.

The therapist can provide reassurance during such periods by helping the patient confront the realities of disease while acknowledging the desire to ignore them. It is also important for the therapist to help reframe feelings about medical treatment "failure," to reconceptualize the notion of "failure" for a person living with chronic infection, and to help the patient move toward a revised health action plan as soon as energy returns. Focusing on activities and short-term goals helps the patient achieve some sense of control in what can otherwise feel like an overwhelming situation.

THE COUNSELOR AS LIAISON

Family and Friends
Given the nature of HIV illness, friends, partners, and family members are often involved in clients' attempts to manage their feelings and their lives. In addition to providing support for these people, counselors can help patients cope with inevitable family pressures and dynamics.

Some clients may have suffered a lifetime of discrimination and abuse from family members as a result of their sexual orientation and/or addiction. Or, steadfast lovers and friends may find themselves snubbed by family members and suddenly excluded from decision making. Because the desires of clients with AIDS sometimes conflict with the competing interests and expectations of families, friends, lovers, and health care providers, therapists may find themselves repeatedly playing the role of mediator.

Therapists can also assist families overburdened by the demands of home care, particularly when illness has progressed to dementia. Emotionally, the family needs to recognize its limits while working through grief and guilt. The therapist can also play a concrete role in marshaling the aid and services of outside social resources.

Working with Physicians
While active participation in one's medical care is essential, it is also highly challenging. Therapists can have an important role in facilitating clients' decision-making processes. For many patients, the concept of developing relationships with medical providers and becoming an active member of the medical team is a foreign one. This is especially true for poor patients who typically receive care at emergency rooms and clinics where frequent staff rota-

tion and institutional insensitivity is common. Moreover, physicians who are unaccustomed to patient involvement in treatment decisions may resist or resent patients' desires for participation. Therapists can often teach clients to assert themselves more effectively without being considered abrasive. Role playing is a useful technique for helping patients develop these skills.

In the following case, the counselor succeeded in helping his client obtain better medical care by reducing the friction that had characterized the client's previous interactions with health care providers.

CASE #2: Jim

Jim was a 26-year-old man with HIV-related symptoms, but no opportunistic infections, and a history of psychiatric hospitalizations, including suicide threats. Because of the negative behaviors toward his physician (as well as the medical office staff) and volunteers with the local AIDS service organization, Jim often did not obtain either the medical care or the emotional support he needed. He was demanding of his counselor as well, often raging at him and at life in general. He would show up late for appointments and then become upset when the counselor ended the sessions on time.

Jim's counselor provided consistent guidelines and was extremely patient, not responding defensively to personal verbal attacks. He realized that his role was to "be there" for Jim, regardless of how Jim behaved. Although it was Jim's own behavior that turned others off, he experienced rejections wherever he turned.

The counseling sessions proved a safe place in which Jim could express a wide range of emotions, including intense fear, rage, and despair. Over time he gained insight into the negative consequences of his own, often inappropriate, behavior, which he was able to modify. Consequently, Jim was able to receive better medical care. The need for psychiatric intervention was reduced, and Jim's physical, as well as social, functioning improved.

LATE-STAGE ILLNESS

Coping with Chronic Illness and Physical Decline

As HIV infection progresses and the body deteriorates, many young patients report feeling "trapped" in a 70- or 80-year-old body. Unlike the elderly, whose peers share anecdotes about physical changes, young people with HIV infection have few places where they can talk freely about new infections, lesions, increasing levels of fatigue, loss of libido, or hair loss. Support groups can provide a useful and safe environment for such exchanges.

Increasing impairment and dependence on others are often significant sources of distress for individuals during later stages of HIV infection. By helping clients develop new activities and goals, the therapist can be instrumental in helping clients preserve their sense of purpose and self-sufficiency. A wide variety of volunteer, leisure, personal growth, or advocacy activities can accommodate disability and can provide HIV-infected individuals with a sense of usefulness. Clients can be taught strategies that can be applied to various situations likely to arise during the course of the disease. For example, as clients get sicker, they might be encouraged to focus less on new treatment modalities and more on relaxation, dealing with family members, completing unfinished business, and making legal and/or financial arrangements.

The illnesses and deaths of other people with HIV infection among one's immediate circle of friends and family can be overwhelmingly frightening at times. Such experiences evoke anticipatory grief and feelings of loss as HIV-infected clients confront the possibility of their own diminishing health. The therapist's office is often the only place the HIV-infected client has in which to truly grieve, and the therapist is the only one trusted to witness and validate the client's loss. Clients need to grieve for the loss of the healthy person they used to be, and for the loss of their dreams and aspirations. HIV is a disease of loss after loss, constantly challenging good therapists to uncover new sources of hope for clients.

Talking About Death and Dying

Therapists can support their clients' decisions about how they want to be cared for and where, how, and when they wish to die. Such decisions are complex. Since physicians may not always address these issues, the therapist may be the only person willing to help weigh options and clarify desires. It is common for people to put off decisions about wills, living wills, "do not resuscitate" orders, durable power of attorney, guardianship of children, and funeral arrangements because making those decisions requires confronting—and accepting—the emotional and practical realities of the end of life. Therapists can help by raising important issues, by directing clients toward local legal resources, and by supporting all of these efforts.

As death approaches, the patient's goals may shift. Initially, there may be hope for recovery or stabilization but as HIV progresses, perspective often changes. The person may hope to live through this summer, until a child visits, or until a cherished project is completed. Later, hope may be invested in the activities of friends and family who will survive, or in a peaceful death that occurs in a manner consistent with the client's wishes.

If the individual is religious, he or she may focus on eternal life and eventually reuniting with friends or family. As perspective shifts, the therapist can assist the client to redirect his or her energy to the goals and activities that matter most.

Clients can maintain a sense of control by continuing to be involved in the decisions of family and friends, by learning systematic desensitization and self-hypnosis to decrease pain and side effects of drugs, and by continuing to make small decisions, such as which vein should be selected for I.V.s, when to be bathed, and where flowers should be placed. One of the most critical decisions that remains within the client's domain is the place of dying. Therapists can and should support dying clients and their families in making such plans and decisions.

Although there is no single "correct" way to approach dying clients, an open mind is crucial. At the end of life, clients are often quite acutely aware of their needs, strengths, and weaknesses. While therapists may find themselves becoming more passive, their very presence is significant. Experienced therapists sometimes refer to their role at this stage as that of a witness.

Friends and family frequently withdraw during the end stages of disease for a variety of reasons, ranging from feelings of inadequacy and guilt to fears of contamination. Patients who are dying also withdraw. It is a way of letting go. Families and friends need to know that withdrawal is normal and natural, and should not take offense. Communication patterns during terminal illness are often complicated by past family dynamics in which unresolved tensions aggravate an already tense situation. The therapist's assistance at the bedside, both in hospital and at home, can be helpful in these situations.

Sometimes, by making it safe to face the reality of death, the counselor can actually help the client find meaning and purpose in whatever time is left, as is illustrated in the following case.

CASE #3: Joan

Joan was a 44-year-old single mother who had late-stage illness and three children—ages 5, 8, and 18. When the counselor first became involved with Joan, she was still in good health. By this time, however, the counselor began to feel overwhelmed, feeling that there was nothing she could do for Joan anymore.

The counselor's peer supervisor helped her to realize that she had, in fact, taken on Joan's feelings of hopelessness and despair. Moreover, because of significant illness progression, the counselor was also experiencing anticipatory grief. There were still a number of things to be attended to and a number of ways in which the counselor could still help Joan.

Although formal arrangements had been made for the children, Joan had never talked with them, or anyone, about her death. By asking about her worst fears and concerns, the counselor created opportunities for Joan to talk about death and dying. Eventually, they discussed some of the concrete issues that needed to be decided. These sessions brought Joan tremendous relief. She had avoided talking about her own death because she was afraid of seeming as if she had given up; she also felt that somehow, "talking about it would make it happen."

When she was ready to discuss her thoughts about dying with her children, the counselor helped her devise appropriate strategies. Joan spoke with her oldest child, from whom she had felt alienated, first. The counselor was involved during the discussions with the younger children. Not only did Joan appreciate the counselor's support during those talks, she was also pleased that the children had formed a connection with the counselor that could be helpful after she died. The counselor reassured Joan that she would indeed be there to help the children through that period.

Counseling led Joan to make a videotape for the younger children that would tell them some of the things she wanted to say but felt they were too young to understand. On videotape, she told them who she was as a person, what her hopes and dreams for them were, advised them about coping with life's challenges, and emphasized that they should "always believe in themselves." This project provided Joan with renewed strength and vigor, and indeed, interest in her life.

Saying Good-Bye

Saying good-bye is extremely difficult and is something that even experienced counselors tend to avoid. Nevertheless, good therapists often encourage their dying clients to consider whether they feel that anything remains left unsaid or undone. The therapist must ask the same question of himself or herself. Sometimes it is useful to ask a dying person, "Why are you still holding on, when it's obvious you're suffering a great deal?" Their answer may be instrumental in helping in the letting go process.

To be helpful to the dying client, the therapist must be emotionally present in the relationship. Interactions with the client, however, should not be used to work through the therapist's own unresolved grief. Such issues should be raised and dealt with through peer supervision or peer support groups. Therapists working with AIDS patients can find the work as rewarding as it is challenging, but they need support. Therapists also need to recognize that they are human and must find ways to schedule breaks in their work so that they can continue to be effective.

REFERENCES

Atkinson JH, Grant I, Kennedy CJ, Richman DD, Spector SA, McCutchan A. Prevalence of psychiatric disorders among men infected with human immunodeficiency virus: a controlled study. *Archives of General Psychiatry*. 1988 45:859-864.

Beckett A, Shenson D. Suicide risk in patients with human immunodeficiency virus infection and AIDS. *Harvard Review of Psychiatry*. 1993;1:27-35.

Bialer PA, Wallack JJ, Snyder SL. Psychiatric diagnosis in HIV-spectrum disorders. *Psychiatric Medicine*. 1991:9(3):361-375.

Caldwell SA, Burnham RA, Forstein M. *Therapists on the Front Line: Psychotherapy with Gay Men in the Age of AIDS*. Washington, D.C.: American Psychiatric Press, Inc; 1994.

Dilley JW, Ochitill HN, Perl M, Volberding P. Findings in psychiatric consultations with patients with acquired immune deficiency syndrome. *American Journal of Psychiatry*. 1985;142:82-86.

Erikson EH. *Childhood and Society*. New York: W.W. Norton & Co.;1959.

Frierson RL, Lippmann SB. Suicide and AIDS. *Psychosomatics*. 1988;29: 226-231.

Green J, McCreaner A. *Counselling in HIV Infection and AIDS*. Cambridge, MA: Blackwell Scientific Publications; 1989.

Jung CG. The Stages of Life. In: Read H, Fordham M, Adler, G, eds. *The Collected Works of C.G. Jung: The Structure and Dynamics of the Psyche*. New York: Pantheon Books;1960.

Kizer KW, et al. AIDS and suicide in California (letter). *Journal of the American Medical Association*. 1988;260:1881.

Markowitz J, Rabkin JG, Perry SW. Treating depression in HIV-positive patients (editorial review). *AIDS*. 1994;8:403-412.

Marzuk P, Tierney H, Tardiff K, et al. Increased risk of suicide in persons with AIDS. *Journal of the American Medical Association*. 1988;259:1333-1337.

Mulleady G. *Counselling Drug Users About HIV and AIDS*. Cambridge, MA: Blackwell Scientific Publications; 1992.

Nichols S. Psychosocial reactions of persons with acquired immunodeficiency syndrome. *Annals of Internal Medicine*. 1985;103:765-767.

Ostrow DG, Monjan A, Joseph J, et al. HIV-related symptoms and psychological functioning in a cohort of homosexual men. *American Journal of Psychiatry*. 1989;146:737-742.

Rabkin JG, Remien RH, Katoff L. Resilience in adversity among AIDS long-term survivors. *Hospital and Community Psychiatry*. 1993;44:162-167.

Rabkin JG, Rabkin, R, Harrison W, Wagner G. Effect of imipramine on mood and enumerative measures of immune status in depressed patients with HIV illness. *American Journal of Psychiatry*. 1994;151:516-523.

Satz P, Miller E, Visscher B, Van Gorp W, D'Elia LF, Dudley J. Changes in mood as a function of HIV status: a 3-year longitudinal study. International Conference on AIDS, Stockholm, June 12-16, 1988. Abstract no. 8598.

Thomas, M. The Eriksonian Model as a Framework for the Psychosocial Assessment of the HIV-Seropositive Individual, unpublished doctoral dissertation. Teacher's College, Columbia University, NY, NY, 1994.

Tross S, Hirsch DA, Rabkin B, Berry C, Holland JC. Determinants of current psychiatric disorder in AIDS spectrum patients. Proceedings of the Third International Conference on AIDS. Washington, D.C., 1987.

Williams JBW, Rabkin JG, Remien RH, Gorman JM, Ehrhardt A. Multidisciplinary baseline assessment of homosexual men with and without human immunodeficiency virus infection. II. Standardized clinical assessment of current and lifetime psychopathology. *Archives of General Psychiatry*. 1991;48:124-130.

Winiarski M. *AIDS-Related Psychotherapy*, New York: Pergamon Press; 1991.

13

TASKS FOR FRIENDS AND FAMILY

COMMENT

Relationships, while enriching, are often complicated. When a friend or loved one becomes ill, such complications can become overwhelming. Those who care for and about people with AIDS need to recognize the double-edged effects of sympathy and the realities of social awkwardness and embarrassment; they need to set limits and to accept the possibility of emotional withdrawal. Most of all, they need to be ready to face the intense passions—their own and their loved one's—evoked by HIV infection, such as envy, guilt, fear, and all-encompassing anger. For the person whose friend, son, daughter, sibling or life partner is ill, balancing ambivalent and often multilayered feelings can be a complex and challenging—and ultimately enriching—task.

Human friendships and attachments are complex by their very nature and in the best of circumstances. In the context of HIV, unresolved issues, inconsistencies, and contradictions become magnified, and a host of new issues, specific to this chronic illness, often emerge. This chapter focuses on potential difficulties and novel challenges that may arise among people affected by AIDS, and describes strategies that have been found helpful.

The term "family" refers to those people one turns to for help and guidance, and who willingly accept these roles. While the term usually refers to one's biological "family of origin," including parents, siblings, and children, it may include other relatives, such as grandparents, cousins, aunts, and uncles. For many people with HIV illness, family consists of biologically unrelated peers in their community. Gay men often have "reconstituted" families, including other gay men and lesbians, with whom the standard holidays are regularly celebrated. Former drug users may have reconstituted families consisting of people they have met through 12-step programs and support groups. And for those who are ill, family may include buddies and caregivers to whom they have grown attached. A broad but useful definition of family as "all those people who decide to go through this experience with their loved one" was given in *The AIDS Caregiver's Handbook* (Eidson, 1988, p 91).

Several of the issues addressed in this chapter were thoughtfully explored by a man named Richard who was himself living with AIDS amidst a crowd of friends and family. We turn to his voice throughout this discussion.

HUMANS ARE SOCIAL CREATURES

Some people live their lives as loners, with only superficial ties to those around them. Most, however, are connected in some ways to other people. If someone develops HIV illness, everyone in his or her life becomes somehow involved. Even those who deliberately divorce themselves from their HIV-positive friends or relatives are "involved." Richard explained this phenomenon, "Those who willfully look in other directions can only be said to speak loudly in their silences...."

In a commentary about friendships and AIDS, Richard began with this observation:

> Contrary to the standard media image of the solitary AIDS sufferer, AIDS happens not only to an individual, but to the people who surround him or her as well. This group of caretakers may be made up of a traditional family. More often it's composed of a more diverse [group]. Sometimes it's a combination of family and friends, often leading to struggles and tensions. Certainly the group includes doctors, nurses, therapists, support group members, homecare health attendants, neighbors and tenants of a building, even strangers, who for various reasons volunteer to come face to face with this devastating illness. For AIDS is happening everywhere. AIDS has changed the world, there's no going back. The catastrophe has already happened. Cruelly perhaps, even those fortunate enough to survive the pandemic physically will also "live with AIDS" for the rest of their lives....

The tasks of friends and family are not simple, in part because they often entail novel situations and roles. Basically, the "job description" is "to stand by, to do whatever can be done, to comfort...." (Thomas, 1992, p 48).

AT THE BEGINNING

When people first learn that a friend or family member has HIV illness, they may err in the magnitude of their reactions in two ways: they may avoid the person (for whatever reason) or they may be overly solicitous. Although the former is sometimes expected, surprisingly, the latter also occurs. Then, ironically, instead of having to deal with rebuff from family members, the patient may need to ward off excessive attention and constant queries. It may require some practice and mutual adjustment to reach a comfortable balance between expressing interest and concern and being intrusive. A common mistake made by those close to an HIV-positive person is conferring "patient" status prematurely.

A few people, for whatever reason, do seem to withdraw their friendship upon disclosure of HIV-positive status. Although this is a hurtful response, most HIV-positive people eventually conclude that true friends are those on whom one can depend, especially in hard times.

Breaking the News

The complexities of disclosing one's HIV-positive status and techniques for doing so have been covered elsewhere in this book (Chapters 7 and 12). The announcement itself is usually greeted with varying degrees of shock and disbelief, depending on the listener's level of surprise. Particularly among unsuspecting parents, there may be tears accompanied by guilt and anger. The "discloser" should be composed and self-possessed when imparting the information. If he or she bursts into tears, the despair will be contagious, and the situation will be viewed as a calamity. Anticipating the "listener's" fears and preparing answers will help both parties maintain control and perspective. Questions should always be encouraged.

A really graceful response of a loved one, upon hearing the news, ideally, would be to hug the person and say in effect, "I love you and I'll help in any way I can." Most relatives and friends, however, experience some degree of shock and need time to adjust to the news, as did the HIV-positive person him- or herself. It is certainly also appropriate to express sadness, but not to fall apart, demanding comfort and consolation. In fact, the likelihood of the latter reaction actually keeps quite a few HIV-positive people from telling their parents, since this anticipated additional burden is more than they feel ready to handle.

Everyone Needs Support

Everyone needs support when someone he or she cares about is in trouble. Friends and family are understandably upset, sad, angry, and distraught when they learn a loved one has HIV illness. However, when the HIV-positive person announces the news, or starts to become seriously ill, or is first hospitalized, he or she should not be obliged to comfort others. Although some may find the role of "comforter" helpful in dealing with distress, as a rule, the focus should more appropriately be placed on the needs of the infected person. One man, wise to the experience of illness as a result of numerous hospitalizations, ordered a t-shirt with "THIS IS ABOUT ME" printed across the chest. He wore it in the hospital to emphasize to his friends that they weren't supposed to turn to him for consolation, entertainment, or diversion in this setting. In any event, the person hearing the news should bear in mind that the individual always most in need of support is the HIV-positive person him- or herself.

"Being There"

In addition to expressing concern and interest in the infected person's health, it is important for friends to express reassurance that the relationship will remain unchanged. People need to know that their friendship is valued, that their company is appreciated, and that they still have interests and activities in common with their friends. Even if there have been lapses in the past, friends should make an extra effort at this time to be reliable and dependable.

Discretion

A promise of confidentiality is paramount. Anyone who is close enough to the individual to be informed of his or her HIV-positive status should not betray that trust. Being HIV-positive still carries significant societal stigma. Friends and relatives should not gossip about the person's condition with mutual friends, unless there is a compelling reason to do so (e.g., inappropriate and self-destructive behavior on the part of the infected person).

Living a Normal Life

Diagnosis of HIV infection does not, and should not, require immediate changes in one's routine. Friends and family can help to preserve normalcy by maintaining enjoyable customs, patterns, and shared activities. No lifestyle changes may be necessary for several years at least, and in this context, sameness is often reassuring.

A future orientation is an essential part of normal living. The HIV-positive person should be supported in his or her future plans rather than warned of impending decline. If people with HIV look forward to returning to school, getting professional training, or seeing their children grow up, the anticipation itself may be pleasurable.

One of the key ways in which friends and other loved ones maintain normalcy is to treat people as people, not as patients. One man explained the difficulties and discomforts caused by HIV-negative people when they insisted, no matter how lovingly, on relating to him as a person with a disease:

> With people who are negative, people from the "outside," I have to be careful with everything I say because either they're going to get hysterical about something or misinterpret whatever I say as having a drastic meaning. I can never just say anything lightly. My HIV status is always part of their agenda. They can never look at me without seeing AIDS, the medical condition.
>
> For example, the daughter of one friend who passed away kept wanting to come see me and bring me food. Last time she said that, I said, "Damn it, let's just go out for dinner, or I'll cook something." And she said, "Well, do you think you could, physically?" And I said, "I don't know why not, I do it every other night of the week."
>
> People start to cling, and that is uncomfortable. It's like clothes that stick to you. Sticking is uncomfortable. I find myself reassuring people too often, "It's okay I have AIDS. Don't worry about it, I can handle it." My feeling is, "Don't keep reminding me. I feel good today, so don't remind me I may feel bad tomorrow."

WHEN ILLNESS BECOMES CHRONIC

Setting Boundaries, Defining Limits, Giving Cues

Although one should not suddenly be transformed into a "patient" simply by virtue of informing others of one's HIV-positive status, eventually adjustments become necessary. Relationships are bound to change as a person becomes ill. Nevertheless, acknowledging the increasing infirmity and consequent dependence of the ill person can be very difficult for all concerned.

Many people don't know how they should act or what they should say. In fact, one reason people tend to avoid their ill friends is simple social awkwardness. Embarrassment probably motivates a lot of behavior. It may help for the HIV-positive person to give straightforward instructions and just tell people what is needed. Friends and family might also ask what is wanted or simply express their discomfort by saying something like, "I feel awkward talking with you about this, but...." If offers to help are regularly rejected, a friend might say, "I'd like to be helpful but it seems I'm always being turned down. How could I be most useful?" Most of the time, it is more effective to ask than to guess or to remain silent.

Richard's effort at writing about friendships was inspired by a friend. He shouted at him:

> "So you have AIDS—what do you want me to do about it?" That really left me wondering. What do I want other people to do? What can they do? I never really thought about that before. This episode happened just last year, so it was 4 or 5 years into my illness before I really began to wonder what it is that other people can do. I guess for all those years before, I and all the people around me were sort of on automatic, just doing things we thought we should be doing, but not really thinking about it. That question, you know, created a lot of distance between my best friend and me. But it also made me realize that I hadn't been thinking enough about what it was I needed or wanted done and what it was that other people could or would actually do.

Expectations should be, and almost invariably are, different for different people. Some relatives and friends may be totally available, both emotionally and physically. Others may have limited resources to share. Those who cannot be 100% involved can still have meaningful interactions and relationships. And regardless of how available or involved people can be, general good manners like courtesy and respect for privacy and independence may be expected from everyone.

When a loved one becomes ill, we may believe that, even as love may be unconditional, so our willingness and availability to help, or to simply "be there," also ought to be unconditional. In real life, however, this is rarely possible, even for partners or other household members. Not only do most people have obligations that cannot be indefinitely suspended, but also as the person with HIV illness gets sicker, it is nearly impossible for one person to provide all necessary care. The notion of "doing it all" alone is neither wise nor feasible.

Sometimes in a crisis, friends or family make offers of assistance that they later regret. In the long run, however, it is kinder to set reasonable boundaries than to renege on impossible promises or to resent the all-consuming demands of the caregiver role. It is often helpful to ask specific questions before offering assistance with a proposed task: How much time will it take? How often? Will there be a back-up? Reliability is essential in this context: Deliver on all promises, but promise only that which can be delivered.

Staying the Course

While friends are cautioned against total sacrifice to the care of the sick person, it is also a particularly painful time to disappear. In the face of illness progression, the person with AIDS especially needs to feel others can be counted on. One man with long-term chronic illness said,

> My boyfriend did this really weird disappearing act. He just faded. Finally I cornered him once, and he let me know that I was getting to be kind of a drag to be with, and that's a quote. And I said, "Honey, AIDS is a kind of major drag. I couldn't agree with you more." He just couldn't handle it emotionally. The odd thing is that he's [HIV] positive. He's not running for fear of contagion. What he's afraid of is seeing what will happen to him.

AIDS is a terrible disease. Friends and loved ones who continue to share themselves with the infected person should be appreciated and cherished. For those who stay the course, there may be heartbreak, but there won't be regret.

How to Help

Either during an acute illness, as in the period after hospital discharge, or when illness becomes chronic, the issue of providing practical assistance arises. While a few people become dependent prematurely, more often the converse is the case: People may truly need help but don't want to acknowledge or accept it. For friends, this situation is perplexing: Do you wait for someone to ask for help? Do you ask whether he or she wants help? Do you simply plunge in and help without being invited? Interfering with a person's autonomy and privacy in order to address perceived unmet needs is again a question of boundaries. What must be clarified is exactly whose needs are being addressed. In general, friends should make clear that they are not "taking over," but are merely doing whatever legwork the ill person indicates is important to him or her.

If financial resources are available, the option of hiring someone to carry out routine tasks, such as cleaning, laundry, and shopping should be considered. Alternatively, larger communities with local community-based AIDS organizations may offer buddy programs: Volunteers provide help, usually on a limited basis. In several of the AIDS epicenters, highly specialized services are available to PWAs (persons with AIDS) for the asking: free meals delivered to the home on a day's notice, dog walking or other animal care, and even weekly delivery of donated flowers (Los Angeles).

Such assistance is sometimes more palatable if it is proposed on a trial basis. And, it is sometimes easier to accept such services from a person being paid to do them than from a friend or partner. Hiring someone is a financial transaction, devoid of emotional baggage, guilt, or obligation. Moreover, if routine tasks are taken care of, friends can visit to chat and be companionable instead of running errands.

Less intimate friends may be very helpful in late-stage illness by letting it be known that they are available for specific tasks. For example, one friend with a car and a flexible work schedule might be able to provide transportation to the physician's office or clinic. Another may like to cook and deliver some meals.

The person with HIV illness also must think about setting boundaries. With good intentions, people may call too often, visit too much, or stay too long. When one is ill with pain or nausea or fever, it may be more restful to be alone. This message can be communicated gracefully, without offending, and is entirely appropriate.

Responding to Withdrawal

A difficult situation may develop when the sick person stops communicating with others. He or she may not answer the phone or return messages, may not permit visitors, may not open the door if visitors do come, or may ask visitors to leave after 5 minutes. Alternatively, the sick person may just lie in bed, remaining silent and remote.

One such man, with many chronically unpleasant but not immediately life-threatening conditions, became increasingly detached and withdrawn, staying in bed with the blinds drawn for days at a time. When his only visitor came, he said, "People only make me feel worse. I don't want to be a pet gerbil. I need to be alone. I don't want to see anybody because it doesn't give me any pleasure anyway and I'll only hurt them. I don't want attachments. I don't want commitments. I don't want ties. I feel lonelier around people, and their expectations are annoying."

What should friends and relatives do when the patient withdraws? Where is the line between appropriate concern (about possible neglect of nutrition, medication, and other essential matters) and invasion of privacy? The image of being a "pet gerbil" is disturbing because it does approximate much of the friend's or relative's role as the HIV-positive person gets sicker. The caregiver provides food and drink and a clean, warm, safe "nest." If independence is an unresolved issue for the sick person, it is easy to understand the distaste he or she may feel for the entire situation.

There is no simple or single correct response to withdrawal. Each patient or friend has to work this out individually, and again, consider exactly whose needs are being served. In general, friends should think about the stage of illness, and the presence or absence of other people in the patient's life.

During episodes of acute illness, when medical care is being provided in a hospital or home setting, friends can offer companionship, affection, support, and reassurance. Difficulties more commonly arise when the ill person has progressed to a phase when they are seldom well. During this time, he or she may have reduced energy, mobility, and stamina due to persistent symptoms, such as neuropathy, pain, nausea, and diarrhea.

Late-stage illness commonly entails a gradual detachment of interest and investment in the world in general. Social attachments may be limited to a few central people. These people may be long-time intimates, or they may be newly arrived in the life of the patient, such as home attendants or nurses.

The question for friends and those outside the immediate household then becomes how aggressively to pursue contact. If there is a partner living with the ill person, he or she may be able to provide guidance. More often, the patient lives alone. In deciding how aggressively to pursue contact, one might consider who else is on the scene. If the sick person has a few close friends who are permitted to communicate and visit, check medication, and replenish food supplies, then it might be best to step aside. If, on the other hand, the sick person is not in regular touch with anyone else, it is probably appropriate to be more insistent, even pushy, about stopping by from time to time.

Responding to Cognitive Impairment

As time passes, some HIV-positive people develop problems with memory, mental quickness, and verbal fluency. For most, the changes are mild and never interfere with daily life. There are some people, however, who develop major cognitive problems, which may be accompanied by difficulty with balance and motor coordination as well as increasing apathy and withdrawal. Personality changes also may be observed. While clear-cut AIDS-related dementia is most often seen very late in illness, it can develop earlier in the disease when people are still being cared for at home. When it does, it can create major management problems for friends and family: When to insist on visiting? When to take over responsibility for tasks like grocery shopping? When to provide supervision for meals and medication?

This situation, when it happens, is burdensome, difficult and discouraging. Help can be provided by organizing, simplifying, and structuring daily activities and tasks for the sick person. Increasing supervision may be called for, which is almost always best handled with the assistance of home aides. Sharing responsibilities with other friends and relatives in this difficult situation also helps.

Visiting

A very ill person may prefer silence. Conversation, or even listening, may simply require too much effort. The author of a classic book about the end of life wrote, "This is the time when the television is off. Our communications then become more nonverbal than verbal. The patient...may just hold our hand and ask us to sit in silence. Such moments of silence may be the most meaningful communications for people....our presence may just confirm that we are going to be around until the end" (Kubler-Ross, 1969, p 113). Although some people forbid visits when they are in the hospital or at home ill, most appreciate the reassurance that they have not been abandoned. At such times, it is prudent to limit visits to 10 or 15 minutes. Or, the visitor may sit and read a book while the patient dozes. Sometimes, when the end is very near, the visitor can do more to support a devoted partner or the family than can be done for the patient.

Mutual Obligations

A Chinese fortune cookie advised, "In order to have a friend, you must be one." Most emotionally healthy adults recognize the mutuality of relationships. In the face of illness, however, that point sometimes can become obscured. While friends and family must respect the privacy and dignity of the person who is ill, HIV isn't a license to become a prima donna. The HIV-positive person needs to be reasonable about his or her demands of others, or the consequence may be eventual disintegration of the support system.

Maintaining a balanced relationship can become increasingly difficult as illness progresses. This was illustrated by a case of two men who had been together for many years. One was hospitalized with a serious condition for 3 weeks. He was on a special AIDS unit with an attentive and caring staff. The other supported them both, living and working at a job on the other side of town. The patient asked, expected, and demanded that his partner come across town before work to help him dress and get to the bathroom, although hospital staff were available to help. The partner was then to go to work, returning directly to the hospital in the evening to keep the patient company. At 9 or 10 P.M., the partner could then go home, which was across town. There were hardly any other visitors. The partner felt obligated, and exhausted himself trying to fulfill these unreasonable expectations. When the time for hospital discharge approached, the patient refused to have home attendants because he didn't like strangers. The partner became increasingly doubtful of his ability to manage with this very sick, frightened patient. His neediness seemed insatiable. The patient called a therapist, declaring, "I think I should commit suicide. I'm too much of a burden for Joe." Joe, the partner, in turn, called and said, "I have burn-out. I can't go on. He'll have to go back to the hospital." Clearly, the inability of either to set limits produced a mutually devastating situation that was resolved when an outsider said simply, "Home care will begin tomorrow." The situation eased and both relaxed. When the patient died soon thereafter in the presence of his partner (and home attendant), both were calm at the end.

It is in the interest of everyone to be reasonable and measured both in what is asked for and in what is given. This is hardly easy for some people even when times are good. In crisis, it can be incredibly difficult. But it is essential.

COMMON EMOTIONAL RESPONSES

Sympathy: Supportive or Patronizing?

Expressing sympathy, by word or actions, appears the right thing to do, the socially expected response to someone's illness, the polite reaction in a social situation. It isn't always communicated or perceived that way, however. As Richard explained:

> Sympathy, I realized, had become a double-edged sword. I thought I wanted it and had always without much thought considered it to be one of the natural virtues, but once I became seriously ill and the recipient of an enormous amount of sympathy, I began to detect something pacifying, something that seemed to promote in me a kind of passivity. Instead of murmuring expressions of sorrow and care, I began to long for people who would tell me to get off my ass and get over myself. I no longer wanted to be treated like a sick person. Such treatment only fed any nagging lethargy and death wish that I, as anyone else, might have. Where were the friends who had refused to indulge me?

Richard was on target. Sympathy is a "two-edged" response. Its positive side is intuitively obvious, but what about its negative aspects? How are feelings of pity, sympathy, empathy, "feeling for and feeling with" distinguished? When is sympathy used as a divider or means of distancing ("You're sick and I'm not"), or as a way to imply altered status ("you poor thing"), or as a way to avoid doing anything? How can one *not* express sympathy for someone who is loved and so sorely tried? "Tough love" or indifference seems callous and unfeeling. The individuals involved, the stage of illness, and physical condition will determine how an appropriate balance can be achieved.

Anger

Richard told this story:

> "So you have AIDS, what do you want me to do about it", shouted my best friend at me late one night. We had been having dinner with another guy, a boy with AIDS who was not doing well but who laughed at all his problems and treated his illness as a big joke. My best friend laughed with him and egged him on to make more fun of what was a desperately serious situation. I grew more and more depressed and silent in the face of their merriment. As they became drunk, I became furious. After the sick boy had left, my friend and I quarreled bitterly over what seemed to me to be a shockingly callous attitude on his part—he is HIV negative—towards the life and death of close friends. But I also felt a certain gratitude when he shouted at me his fury and exasperations. Ah, I thought, at last some truth telling. I had minded less his anger at me for being ill, which contained within it a germ of compassion, than his refusal to express his anger. The bored, polite sympathy he offered me had seemed false because I knew he found the whole subject dreary and tiresome, and had no real interest in the details.

Those who spend time with people living with AIDS know that the latter are often angry. Friends or relatives may, on occasion, become targets, just by being there, although the anger is characteristically an existential rage about the injustice of losing one's life. In studies of AIDS long-term survivors, comparatively low rates of clinical depression or anxiety were observed; the predominant emotion elicited and reported was anger (Rabkin et al, 1993). Three-quarters of the men interviewed frequently felt very angry. Among the more eloquent responses was this one, given by a man more than 3 years after his AIDS diagnosis: "AIDS has just put a dagger in my life essentially cutting my life in half. I have not reconciled myself to it one bit. To this day I am still in a state of shock that something so awful could happen." Another man, very ill, explained: "My dominant emotion is rage. I'm mostly angry at the sheer frustration of being denied my life." As a rule, such anger can fuel a fierce determination to survive.

Anger can be adaptive in the struggle to engage the best medical care or to become involved as a political activist. Anger at physicians, the government, the loss of friends, is common. Some people are angry at themselves, with more or less reason, for becoming infected. However, if the anger is consistently and exclusively directed at friends, family, and care providers, or the medical system in general, it becomes self-defeating. When possible, volunteer work, political action, letter writing, or marching in demonstrations may represent more productive outlets for the anger that is both intense and inevitable.

What is often overlooked, unrecognized, or denied is the anger of others toward the person with HIV illness. The anticipation of the loss of a child, sibling, parent, or partner can be devastating. One man said, "My brother was angry at me for being HIV-positive and wouldn't talk to me about it. He thought that I, a college graduate, should have known better." More pragmatically, illness causes disappointments, frustrations, irritations, changes of plan. Nobody who has cared about or for a person with AIDS can completely ignore the negative feelings that sometimes arise when the illness interferes with expectations. Acknowledging—and dealing with—the anger is difficult, however, because it seems so petty, so unfair to "blame the victim."

The person with HIV illness also may be slow to recognize this anger in those around him. Richard observed:

> It was actually my support group leader that pointed it out to me. "You know your friends are really angry at you for being sick," he said. I had actually never thought about it consciously, but when he said that, I realized that it explained a whole panorama of feelings and responses and slightly strange awkwardness between me and people that I had not really been able to identify before. You are left with the feeling that people are angry when you're ill and they like you when you're well... and that in turn produces anger in yourself, and the feeling that people will only stick around when you're OK. I also think the anger runs deeper than just irritation over

cancelled plans. I think there's an anger that isn't really rational, but that says, "How could you let this happen to you? How could you bring this unpleasantness into all of our lives?" I had felt some of that towards other people with AIDS, a feeling that it's almost a personal failure on their part. It's not rational or fair and it's certainly not attractive, but it seems very powerful. That kind of anger needs to be thought about and looked at.

The person who is ill may be equally resentful of those who are HIV-negative or still healthy despite HIV infection. This anger is also difficult to acknowledge. When Richard mentioned the issue of other people's anger toward him in his support group, one person countered with a question about his anger at them for being well:

> There is that also, which is another thing that isn't really talked a lot about, which is the terrible resentment I feel towards healthy people. Strangely enough, I have also felt it from other people with AIDS who were doing worse than I was. When I was in the hospital for a diagnostic procedure with people who were doing very badly—and I was thriving—I felt my health was this terrible conspicuous thing that I had to conceal. I'd try to look ill if I could and cough a lot. It was sort of like having feet that were too big, or wild red hair. My health was all over me and I couldn't hide it enough. Anger goes back and forth between people.

It may be particularly difficult for a person living with AIDS to acknowledge angry feelings toward those he or she counts on for companionship, affection and practical help. Friends and family might directly address the fear of jeopardizing their support by reiterating their commitment: "You can count on me anyway, even if you get grouchy or cranky at times, even if I need to take 'time off' when you get impossible." Of course, this has to be true: Reliability is an essential part of "being there" in any meaningful way.

Anger is part of any close human relationship. Illness does not exempt people from the basic courtesies of living with others. If an individual has a legitimate cause to be angry with someone else, such feelings can and should be openly expressed. But what about when friends and family experience anger at a loved one because of his or her illness? How can such feelings, common as they are, be managed? At one time, people believed in the "teapot" theory of emotions: Anger stayed inside unless you released it, like steam from a boiling tea kettle. Only when anger was let out could it be dissipated. Since then, however, it has been observed that expressing anger as soon as it is experienced may actually generate more anger than deferring its expression. Failure to acknowledge angry feelings, on the other hand, may lead to avoidance of the sick friend or relative.

Talking about the situation with someone who has "been there" can usually provide relief. Perspective, humor, and a good listener can be very helpful. And, often, we feel better after we complain: "We had this wonderful weekend planned, and then he got a fever and wouldn't even let me come over to visit."

It may also be helpful to join a support group for partners, parents, or care providers. These are becoming increasingly available as community-based organizations for people with HIV illness have come to recognize the unmet needs of those who care for and about them. Joining such a group is a more formal but sometimes extremely effective way of coping with your role as the friend or relative of someone who is sick.

What about when friends or family are the unwitting targets of rebuff and anger? A visitor, prepared to do errands like groceries and laundry, might be greeted with the words, "I don't feel like having you here or seeing you today." Or, someone who suggests going out to a show might be bitterly attacked with, "You know I'm too tired to sit through something like that." Or you are given a list of 18 things to get at the supermarket and are greeted with annoyance because you got the wrong brand on one of the items. Even when a friend is permitted to help, he or she might encounter criticism for the way in which certain tasks are done.

When this type of reaction occurs occasionally, most can handle it. If it becomes a pattern, however, it is best to approach the problem directly. Otherwise, a repetitive cycle of anger and guilt will begin that will become increasingly difficult to break.

One might say directly, "I'm trying to think of activities we'll enjoy together and you seem upset by that. Tell me what's the matter." Or, "I'm trying to be useful and all I get is attitude. So how can I help you best?" It may be as simple as a financial problem. It may be a reminder of something they used to do with someone else, friend or partner, whom they have lost. No matter what strategy is tried, it is almost always better to try something than to remain feeling miserable, hurt, angry and finally guilty for a lack of graciousness. It is also helpful to remember that anyone who experiences persistent pain, nausea, fever, and fatigue is likely to be cranky at least some of the time.

Calling to confirm a visit, even a scheduled visit, is a good idea. Reframing goals is also helpful. Instead of expecting to be greeted with pleasure, one can be satisfied with the knowledge that the sick person has an adequate supply of food, for example.

Guilt

Surprisingly often, those who are most dedicated, as well as those only peripherally involved, feel some degree of guilt about not having done enough. When a visitor finds the patient sleeping during a dreaded hospital visit, the response may be relief, followed by guilt. Or, an offer to visit may be turned down, again to the relief of the potential visitor. Worst of all, one may feel relief upon the death of a terribly ill patient, especially if his home had been filled with medical equipment, drugs, and attendants around the clock. While most people feel simply terrible for their own reaction, in reality, relief is an appropriate and fairly common response. Once it is understood as an expected and "normal" response, guilt may be manageable.

FRIENDSHIPS AND AIDS

New Friends

Establishing new ties with someone who is ill is complicated for several reasons, regardless of one's own health status. Richard observed,

> I have to hesitate a little bit now when I meet new people with AIDS. I think, "Do I want another friend with AIDS who is probably not going to make it?" It's a hard decision.
>
> Another thing about friends who have AIDS is that [if you also have AIDS] your whole friendship becomes about AIDS. My doctor, your doctor, my pills, your pills, your stomach, my stomach—that kind of talk can fill a whole friendship. It's amazing, you know, I've spent whole days with people like that, and at the end of it you think what a privilege, but also what a horror, sort of.

In one sense, becoming close to someone whose illness is part of them from the outset is less distressing than discovering that a long-time friend or family member is infected, and then witnessing the gradual decline. With someone who is already ill, there is an awareness, at least at some level, that this friendship is likely be time limited.

Love and Devotion

Despite the difficulties that develop in relationships involving at least one person with HIV illness, there is also the possibility of a transformation of devotion to a level of extraordinary intensity and beauty. This may occur when both partners are ill and take turns caring for each other, or when only one person is ill and the other, who could walk away, chooses not to do so.

We talked to two men about their friendship. The first statement is Steven's, a participant in the Long-term Survivor Study who was interviewed in 1990 after he had been ill for a number of years. Steven was asked, "When you were first diagnosed with PCP, was anything or anyone particularly helpful to you at the time?" He answered:

> My friend. I have a friend who is my old college friend and we're spiritually very close. He's just a beautiful man. He was there for me right at the start and has been, ever since. He has dropped all of his plans for his own life in order to help me. Words cannot describe this type of person. I'm sure there are others doing the equivalent in helping people with AIDS, but nobody could have a more dedicated friend than he has been to me.

Later he was asked, "What brings you pleasure now?"

> My relationship with my friend Bill. I think it validates my life. Whatever happens to me, what we've shared and the kind of love that has been

shown me is a privilege that many, many people never know and for which I'm incredibly grateful. I just thank God. It validates everything I've ever done, no matter the disappointments. We have lived to the maximum in terms of a caring relationship. It is special. It marks me now. I have a great deal of pride in the fact that someone would care that much about me.

About a year later, we called for a follow-up interview and discovered that Steven had died 3 months earlier. His friend wrote the following letter: "I can't begin to describe how badly I miss him, how different and odd and new I feel to myself being in this world without him. Losing him, losing that line out into the future which the feeling of an accompanied heart always gives one, has been an even more total erasure than I'd imagined it would be...."

This exchange brings to mind a passage from St. Augustine, writing of his feelings after the death of his childhood friend: "For I felt that my soul and his were one soul in two bodies, and therefore life was a horror to me, since I did not want to live as a half; and yet I was also afraid to die lest he, whom I had loved so much, would completely die"(Confessions, 4.6).

While loss may be a consequence of attachment, most would agree that a life without the experience of intimacy is worse. In the words of Tennyson, "It is better to have loved and lost than never to have loved at all." Perhaps because of the awareness of life's impermanence, the affection between people (at least one of whom has HIV illness) can attain a purity and intensity possibly never before experienced by either. The limits imposed by awareness of impending mortality may permit the expression of an unconditional love that we fear to risk in other circumstances.

REFERENCES

Eidson E, ed. *The AIDS Caregiver's Handbook.* New York: St. Martin's Press; 1988.

Kubler-Ross E. *On Death and Dying.* New York: Macmillan; 1969.

Rabkin J, Remien R, Katoff L, et al. Suicidality in AIDS long-term survivors: what is the evidence? *AIDS Care.* 1993;5:393-403.

Thomas L. *The Fragile Species.* New York: Scribner; 1992.

I

PAYMENT ASSISTANCE

Name of Drug	Marketing Name	Manufacturer	Indication	Phone
Acyclovir	Zovirax	Burroughs Wellcome	Herpes	(800) 722-9294
Aerosolized pentamidine	NebuPent	Fujisawa	PCP prophylaxis	(800) 336-6323
Atovaquone/566c80	Mepron	Burroughs Wellcome	PCP	(800) 722-9294
Ciprofloxacin	Cipro	Miles	Antibiotic	(203) 937-2000
Clarithromycin	Biaxin	Abbott	Antibiotic/MAC	(800) 688-9118
ddC	Hivid	Hoffmann-La Roche	Antiviral	(800) 285-4484
ddI	Videx	Bristol-Myers Squibb	Antiviral	(800) 788-0123
d4T	Zerit	Bristol-Myers Squibb	Antiviral	(800) 788-0123
Erythropoietin/EPO	Procrit	Ortho Biotech	Antianemia	(800) 441-1336 (800) 447-3437
Erythropoietin/EPO	Epogen	Amgen	Antianemia	(800) 272-9376
Filgrastim/G-CSF	Neupogen	Amgen	Antineutropenic	(800) 272-9376
Fluconazole	Diflucan	Pfizer	Antifungal	(800) 869-9979
Foscarnet	Foscavir	Astra	CMV Acyclovir-resistant herpes	(800) 488-3247
Ganciclovir	Cytovene	Syntex	CMV	(800) 444-4200
Interferon alpha-2b	Intron A	Schering-Plough	Kaposi's sarcoma Hepatitis B, C	(800) 521-7157
Interferon alpha-2a	Roferon-A	Hoffmann-La Roche	Kaposi's sarcoma Hepatitis B, C	(800) 443-6676
Itraconazole	Sporanox	Janssen	Antifungal	(800) 544-2987
Octreotide	Sandostatin	Sandoz	Antidiarrheal	(800) 447-6677
Pyrimethamine	Daraprim	Burroughs Wellcome	Toxoplasmosis	(800) 722-9294
Rifabutin	Mycobutin	Adria	MAC prophylaxis	(800) 795-9759
Sargramostim/GM-CSF	Leukine	Immunex	Antineutropenic	(800) 321-4669
Trimethoprim/ sulfamethoxazole TMP/SMZ	Bactrim	Hoffmann-La Roche	PCP prophylaxis	(800) 443-6676
Trimethoprim/ sulfamethoxazole TMP/SMZ	Septra	Burroughs Wellcome	PCP prophylaxis	(800) 722-9294
Zidovudine/AZT	Retrovir	Burroughs Wellcome	Antiviral	(800) 722-9294

Reprinted with permission from: *POZ*. 1994;June-July:77.

II

TIPS ON HOME CARE

KNOW YOUR RIGHTS*

You have the right...

- To be treated with dignity, consideration, and respect.
- To have your personal property treated with respect.
- To receive confidential care within the extent of the law.
- To know what goods and services are available and their cost.
- To be fully informed about your medical condition.
- To be fully informed about your care and changes in your care.
- To participate in the planning of your care.
- To refuse treatment after being fully informed of the consequences.
- To know the names and responsibilities of the people providing care to you.
- To know that you have the right to make a complaint and the procedure for doing so.

KNOW YOUR INSURANCE

Medicaid

The federal government provides this health insurance for those with a low income or with disabilities. Each state also contributes a share (varies by state). In most states, some form of home health care is covered.

Medicare

The provisions of this federal insurance program are standard throughout the country. It is provided for those over 65 years of age or who are "permanently disabled" for more than 2 years. Limited home care is covered.

Private Insurance

Home care coverage varies, depending on the insurance company and your policy. You may be limited to a list of preferred providers.

WHAT TO ASK ABOUT HOME CARE BENEFITS

- What specific services are provided: registered nurse, continuous nursing service, home health aide, physical therapist, social worker?
- Are medications and medical supplies covered?
- Are there restrictions on the amount or cost of services provided?

---

*Adapted from "Client Bill of Rights."
 Visiting Nurse Service of New York.

- Are there co-payments on the services? Do the co-payments end if a specific dollar amount is reached?
- Are there lifetime caps on what the policy covers? Does coverage end if a specific dollar amount is reached?

HOME CARE AFTER HOSPITALIZATION

- Hospitals are responsible for making home care plans as needed. These arrangements are usually made by discharge planners or social work staff, who are obligated to inform you of these plans and answer questions you may have about the arrangements *before* you leave the hospital.
- At the time of discharge, the hospital should provide you with information about the medications and treatments that you will receive once you are home. You should be informed of any follow-up care related to your hospital stay, such as an appointment at the clinic or physician's office.
- You have the right to select a home care agency. Hospitals or physicians may have agreements with particular agencies, but you are not obligated to accept service from any specific agency unless mandated by your insurance carrier.

GENERAL GUIDELINES

- To receive home care services, you must have a physician who is willing to participate in the coordination of your care. Home care agencies may not provide service without a plan of care signed by a physician.
- The agency is obligated to provide services appropriate to your health needs after performing an assessment and negotiating a plan with your physician. If changes in your care plan become necessary, the agency will make those changes in conjunction with your physician and you.
- Once you are accepted as a client by a home care agency, it becomes responsible for meeting your home care needs. If the agency is unable to do so, it should refer you to an agency that can meet your specific needs. (*Example:* If your physician and the agency feel you need occupational therapy to improve your ability to meet personal care needs, but the agency does not provide this service, it must refer you to an agency that can do so, such as an outpatient rehabilitation center.)
- The agency is obliged to provide the type of services prescribed by your physician. The agency is NOT obliged to fulfill specific requests about staff such as gender, age, ethnicity, or smoking habits, although in many cases agencies try to accommodate.
- If a home health aide is assigned to care for you, a registered nurse (RN) from the agency is required to make home visits on a regular basis (such as every other week). The responsibilities of the nurse are to coordinate, to educate, and to supervise the aide in the plan of care.

ADVICE ABOUT HEALTH CARE

- *Don't Expect Perfection.* The first few days at home can be quite upsetting, especially for people who have never had home care services before. The agency should contact you to make visit arrangements, but problems can arise during the initial transition to home care. It may take 3 or 4 days to get the plan of care operating smoothly.

- *Have Contingency Plans.* You can never be guaranteed that assigned staff will arrive, so it is prudent to have back-up coverage (friends or family) just in case.

- *If you are receiving paraprofessional help* (home health aides, housekeepers), don't expect them to meet your every need. Be realistic and tolerant. Try to find people you are comfortable having in your home and who are capable and willing to learn how to help you.

- *The agency should provide* you with the names and telephone numbers of people to call to report problems. Keep this list readily available. Know whom to call if:

   — Someone doesn't arrive as scheduled, or is chronically late.

   — Supplies or equipment do not arrive as scheduled.

   —There are unresolved conflicts with agency personnel.

   If you have a problem with a particular staff person, make complaints to your service coordinator. It is helpful to clearly specify the nature of the problem (e.g., she comes late and/or leaves early; bad technique with catheter; he speaks inappropriately; your personal property is missing; she takes 2 hours to go to the store on the corner; breach of confidentiality). If the problem is not resolved, move up the chain of command. For serious matters that are not resolved, you may complain to the outside group that licenses the agency, usually at the municipal or state level, and request an investigation. Such requests should be reserved for truly serious problems, however, since investigation can consume considerable personnel and financial resources.

- *Don't Be a "Problem Patient."* People who constantly complain about every detail of their care are often identified as "difficult to serve" and may have difficulty obtaining adequate and compassionate service.

III

HEALTH CARE PROXY AND
MEDICAL DIRECTIVE

I _____ residing at _____,
New York, desiring to designate a Health Care Agent and to state my
wishes about my medical treatment, as permitted by New York law, hereby
execute this Health Care proxy and Medical Directive. I expect my family,
physicians and all those concerned with my care to regard themselves as
legally and morally bound to honor my decisions and the decisions made by
my Health Care Agent on my behalf under the authority I have conferred
on my Health Care Agent below.

1. **Appointment of Health Care Agent.** I appoint _____,
currently residing at _____
TELEPHONE ( )_____ my Health Care Agent to act as
provided in Section 2. If for any reason the person I have here designated as
my Health Care Agent is unable or unwilling to so act, I appoint
_____, currently residing at _____,
TELEPHONE ( )_____ my Health Care Agent.

2. **Authority of Health Care Agent.** In the event I become unable to
make my own health care decisions, I authorize my Health Care Agent to
make health care decisions on my behalf, in accordance with my wishes,
including (but not exclusively) decisions regarding my admission to and discharge from health care facilities, the administration of X-rays, tests, exam-
inations, anesthetics, medical and surgical procedures, and decisions about
life-sustaining procedures in accordance with Sections 3 and 4 below. If my
Health Care Agent shall not know my wishes (either because I have not initialed one or more of the circumstances or procedures listed in Sections 3
or 4 or because the matter to be decided is not covered by Sections 3 or 4)
and cannot with reasonable diligence ascertain them, I authorize my Health
Care Agent to make health care decisions on my behalf in accordance
with my best interests.

I authorize, effective immediately, my Health Care Agent to visit me in
any hospital, convalescent home, or other facility where I may be receiving
treatment or care, and to consult with any physicians and other medical personnel who may treat me. I direct that my Health Care Agent be given first
priority in any such visitation, and I instruct that my medical records,
including (but not exclusively) any confidential HIV related information, be
made available to my Health Care Agent as part of any such consultation.
If my Health Care Agent is not a member of my family, I direct that there

be extended to my Health Care Agent all the rights and powers that any parent, spouse, or other relative of mine would have had if I had not signed this Health Care Proxy and Medical Directive.

3. **Wishes regarding the withholding or withdrawal of life-sustaining procedures.** I have initialed below my wishes regarding the withholding or withdrawal of life-sustaining procedures with respect to the following circumstances:

(Initial **ONE OR MORE** of the lines below)

_____ It is my wish that the procedures initialed in Section 4 be withheld or withdrawn if, in the best judgment of my attending physician, I am permanently unconscious.

_____ It is my wish that the procedures initialed in Section 4 be withheld or withdrawn if I have a condition that is likely to cause my death within a short period of time, whether or not such procedures are administered to me.

_____ It is my wish that the procedures initialed in Section 4 be withheld or withdrawn if I have suffered a substantial and irreversible loss of mental functions.

4. **Life-sustaining procedures to be withheld or withdrawn in accordance with Section 3.** It is my wish that the procedures which I have initialed below shall be Withheld or Withdrawn from me under the circumstances I have initialed in Section 3:

(Initial each procedure to be withheld or withdrawn)

_____ invasive diagnostic procedures

_____ cardiopulmonary resuscitation

_____ mechanical respiratory support

_____ dialysis procedures surgery

_____ antibiotics

_____ artificially administered nutrition

_____ artificially administered hydration

_____ any other extraordinary procedures or measures to sustain my life

I request that I be given appropriate treatment to relieve any pain that I might suffer due to the withholding or withdrawal of any life-sustaining treatment.

Notwithstanding the wishes I have expressed in Sections 3 and 4 above, it is my wish that life-sustaining procedures be administered to me if they are necessary to sustain my life for a reasonable period of time in order to enable _____ to be with me before my death.

5. **Other instructions or comments about care I do or do not want (i.e. experimental treatments; preference to die at home; etc.)** _____

_____

_____

_____

6. **Wishes to be honored in absence of Health Care Agent.** If neither person I have designated in Section I to serve as my Health Care Agent is able and willing to so act, I direct that the life-sustaining procedures I have initialed in Section 4 be withheld or withdrawn under the circumstances I have initialed in Section 3.

7. **Release.** As provided by New York law, my Health Care Agent shall not be subject to any liability for making health care decisions in good faith under this Health Care Proxy and Medical Directive, nor shall any health care provider be subject to any liability or be deemed to have engaged in unprofessional conduct for having honored in good faith the health care decisions made by my Health Care Agent under this Health Care Proxy and Medical Directive.

Any third party may act in reliance on a duly executed copy or facsimile of this Health Care Proxy and Medical Directive. Nothing in this Health Care Proxy and Medical Directive shall rescind or otherwise invalidate any gift of all or part of my body I have made pursuant to the Uniform Anatomical Gifts Act.

8. **Duration.** The time period during which this Health Care Proxy and Medical Directive shall be effective, including (but not exclusively) my authorization of the release of confidential HIV related information to my Health Care Agent, shall begin immediately and will continue, unless I revoke it, for the duration of my life.

THIS HEALTH CARE PROXY AND MEDICAL DIRECTIVE, signed this _____ day of _____, 199__.

_____

Each of the undersigned, being eighteen years of age or older, declares that the person who signed this document is personally known to me, that the same person signed this document in my presence, and appears to be of sound mind and acting willingly and free from duress. None of the undersigned is appointed Health Care Agent by this document.

_____ residing at _____

_____

_____ residing at _____

_____

Note: This proxy is valid in New York State only. See your local AIDS service organization to obtain a proxy valid in your state.

INDEX

Rabkin, Judith G.

Good doctors, good patients